Advanced Emergency Medicine Guide

Optimizing Outcomes in Acute and Critical Care Settings

Dr. Jack R. Davis, MD

Copyright © 2024 Dr. Jack R. Davis, MD.
All rights reserved. No part of this publication may be reproduced, stored in a retrieval system, or transmitted in any form or by any means, electronic, mechanical, photocopying, recording, or otherwise, without prior written permission of the publisher, except for brief quotations used in reviews or scholarly works.

Acknowledgements

The journey of writing Advanced Emergency Medicine Guide: Optimizing Outcomes in Acute and Critical Care Settings has been both challenging and immensely rewarding. I am deeply grateful to all those who have contributed to the development and success of this work, and I would like to take this opportunity to acknowledge their invaluable support.

First and foremost, I wish to express my sincere gratitude to my colleagues in emergency medicine, whose clinical expertise, dedication, and passion for patient care have continually inspired me. Throughout my career, I have learned so much from the many talented professionals with whom I have had the privilege of working. This book reflects not only my personal experiences but also the collective wisdom and efforts of the countless individuals in the field of emergency medicine who have contributed to the advancement of best practices in acute and critical care.

I would like to extend my special thanks to the team at MOM Publishers for their professionalism, guidance, and unwavering support throughout the writing and production process. Their attention to detail, commitment to excellence, and belief in the importance of this work were essential in bringing this guide to fruition.

To the patients I have cared for over the years: Your resilience, trust, and courage have shaped my practice and provided me with invaluable lessons that no textbook could offer. Every case has left an indelible mark on my understanding of medicine, and I remain deeply honored to have had the opportunity to care for you.

I am also profoundly grateful to my family and friends for their endless encouragement and understanding during the writing process. Your support has been my anchor, and without your unwavering belief in my work, this project would not have been possible.

Finally, I wish to acknowledge the tireless work of all healthcare professionals who dedicate their lives to improving patient outcomes in acute and critical care settings. This book is for you—those who work day and night in emergency departments, trauma centers, and intensive care units around the world, where every moment counts, and every decision has the potential to save a life.

I hope this guide serves as a valuable resource in helping you navigate the complexities of emergency medicine and, in turn, contributes to better patient care in emergency and critical care environments worldwide.

Dr. Jack R. Davis, MD
Emergency Medicine Specialist

Preface

In the fast-paced world of emergency medicine, healthcare providers are constantly faced with high-stakes scenarios that demand swift decision-making, expert clinical knowledge, and the ability to adapt to rapidly changing patient conditions. Acute and critical care settings are the front lines of medical practice, where lives hang in the balance, and optimal outcomes are dependent on timely, evidence-based interventions. Advanced Emergency Medicine Guide: Optimizing Outcomes in Acute and Critical Care Settings aims to provide clinicians with a comprehensive and practical resource that addresses the challenges faced in these environments.

As an emergency medicine specialist, I have witnessed firsthand the vital role that effective management plays in ensuring the best possible outcomes for patients in critical conditions. Over the years, I have accumulated extensive experience in handling a wide variety of life-threatening emergencies, from trauma and cardiac arrest to respiratory failure and sepsis. This book is a culmination of that experience, designed to provide a structured, user-friendly guide to managing the complexities of acute and critical care in the emergency department.

The goal of this guide is not only to serve as a reference for healthcare providers but also to empower them with the knowledge to make confident, evidence-based decisions when faced with time-sensitive situations. With a focus on optimizing patient outcomes, the book covers a wide range of topics relevant to the emergency medicine field, from advanced life support protocols to the latest advances in trauma and critical care management. It provides clear, concise explanations of complex concepts, accompanied by real-world case studies, clinical pearls, and actionable insights for immediate application in the clinical setting.

Whether you are an emergency medicine physician, a resident, a nurse practitioner, or a paramedic, this guide is designed to meet your needs by providing both foundational knowledge and advanced clinical strategies. By focusing on practical approaches to diagnosis, treatment, and patient care, Advanced Emergency Medicine Guide aims to enhance the clinician's ability to respond effectively to a wide range of emergencies and improve patient outcomes in both acute and critical care scenarios.

The rapidly evolving nature of emergency medicine means that best practices are always changing. With this in mind, this guide is built upon the latest clinical research, guidelines, and expert consensus to ensure that the information provided is both up-to-date and evidence-based. Throughout the book, emphasis is placed on interdisciplinary collaboration and communication, recognizing that the best outcomes in emergency medicine are often achieved through teamwork and coordinated efforts among all members of the healthcare team.

In addition to clinical management, the guide also addresses key topics in patient safety, ethical dilemmas, and the psychological challenges that emergency clinicians may face. The importance of self-care for healthcare providers, resilience, and mental health are included as essential components for maintaining optimal performance in high-stress environments.

Ultimately, the aim of Advanced Emergency Medicine Guide is to equip you with the tools and knowledge needed to navigate the complexities of emergency medicine, optimize patient care, and contribute to the advancement of healthcare outcomes on a global scale.

I hope this book serves as a valuable resource for you throughout your career, whether you're just beginning your journey in emergency medicine or are an experienced practitioner seeking to refine your skills and knowledge. The challenges of emergency care are great, but with the right knowledge and preparation, we can rise to meet them and make a profound impact on the lives of our patients.

Dr. Jack R. Davis, MD
Emergency Medicine Specialist

Advice to Readers

Always prioritize treating the patient based on their symptoms, not solely relying on monitors or laboratory results.

Begin your assessment with a thorough evaluation of the patient, avoiding preconceived notions based on external investigations to prevent diagnostic bias.

A detailed and accurate history is crucial for making the correct diagnosis; errors in history-taking often lead to misdiagnosis.

Abnormal vital signs should never be overlooked, as they offer a more reliable measure of illness severity than visual assessment alone.

Cultivate strong clinical skills to make accurate diagnoses independently, rather than over-relying on laboratory tests. Sharpen your diagnostic acumen to outpace technology.

Ensure consistency among the patient's history, examination findings, clinical diagnosis, and laboratory results. Discrepancies often point to errors, typically in the laboratory, assuming sound clinical judgment.

Guidelines serve as valuable tools but should not restrict your critical thinking or individualized patient care.

Formulate differential diagnoses based on the patient's history and physical examination before reviewing investigation results.

Embrace change and remain open to questioning established protocols. Strive to improve your knowledge, patient care practices, and the functioning of your department.

Pursue academic excellence and contribute to research. The emergency department offers immense, underutilized opportunities for groundbreaking studies.

Acknowledgement
Preface
Advice to Readers
Table of Contents
List of Abbreviations

Table of contents

Chapter 1: Basic Life Support (BLS)

1. Introduction
   - Overview of Basic Life Support (BLS)
   - Importance of Early Intervention

2. Key Components of Basic Life Support (BLS)
   - Chest Compressions
   - Airway Management
   - Breathing Support
   - Defibrillation

3. Overview of BLS Steps
   - Scene Safety and Initial Assessment

- Recognition of Cardiac Arrest
- Activating the Emergency Response System
- Starting CPR
- Automated External Defibrillator (AED) Use

4. Chest Compressions
    - Principles of High-Quality CPR
    - Compression Rate and Depth
    - Complete Recoil and Minimizing Interruptions
    - Compression-Only CPR

5. Airway Management
    - Methods for Opening the Airway
    - Head Tilt-Chin Lift
    - Jaw Thrust
    - Evidence-Based Practices

6. Ventilation and Respiratory Arrest Management
    - Key Components of Management
    - Basic Airway Adjuncts

- Oropharyngeal Airway (OPA)
- Nasopharyngeal Airway (NPA)
- Rescue Breaths Guidelines
- Bag-Mask Ventilation (BMV)
- E–C Clamp Technique
- Steps for Bag-Mask Ventilation

7. Basic Life Support/CPR for Children (Ages 1 Year to Puberty)
    - Child CPR Sequence
    - Key Differences from Adult CPR

Chapter 2: Management of Cardiac Arrest

1. Introduction
    - Overview of Cardiac Arrest Management
    - Role of the Resuscitation Team
    - Activation of Emergency Response System
    - Basic Life Support (BLS) Protocol

2. Initial Management Steps
    - Monitor Cardiac Rhythm

- Establish Venous Access
- Maintain Airway Patency
- Consider Reversible Causes (5Hs and 5Ts)

3. Common Drugs in Cardiac Arrest
   - Adrenaline (Epinephrine)
   - Amiodarone
   - Lidocaine
   - Atropine
   - Dopamine
   - Magnesium Sulfate
   - Medication Administration via Endotracheal Tube

4. Bradyarrhythmias
   - Definition and Symptoms
   - Management of Bradyarrhythmias
   - First-Line Treatment: Atropine
   - Other Treatment Options
   - Chronotropic Agents
   - Transcutaneous and Transvenous Pacing
   - Reversible Causes of Bradycardia
   - Limitations of Atropine

5. Transcutaneous Pacing
    - Procedure for Transcutaneous Pacing
    - Success Indicators
    - Pad Rotation and Patient Comfort

6. Tachyarrhythmias
    - Definition and Initial Management
    - Synchronized Cardioversion and Medical Therapy
    - Identifying Reversible Causes

7. Immediate Post Cardiac Arrest Care for Adults
    - Key Objectives and Post-Resuscitation Goals
    - Ventilation and Oxygenation
    - Treatment of Hypotension
    - Evaluation of Sensorium
    - Therapeutic Hypothermia and Neurological Recovery

8. Cardiac Arrest in Pregnancy
    - Resuscitation Considerations

- Intravenous Access and Positioning
- Airway Management and Defibrillation
- Fetal Monitoring and Perimortem Cesarean Delivery
- Causes of Maternal Arrest

9. Pediatric Cardiac Arrest
   - Resuscitation Protocol and Compression-Ventilation Ratio
   - Defibrillation and Paddle Size Considerations
   - Monitoring and Post-Arrest Care

Chapter 3: Understanding and Managing Anaphylaxis

1. Introduction
   - Overview of Anaphylaxis
   - Organ Systems Involved

2. Diagnostic Criteria for Anaphylaxis
   - Criterion 1: Acute Onset with Skin or Mucosal Involvement

- Criterion 2: Rapid Onset After Allergen Exposure
- Criterion 3: Hypotension Following Allergen Exposure

3. Management of Anaphylaxis
    - Eliminate the Trigger
    - Airway Management
    - Oxygenation
    - Circulation Support
    - Patient Positioning
    - Adrenaline Administration
    - Antihistamines
    - Adjunctive Therapies

4. Observation and Discharge
    - Post-Discharge Considerations

5. Key Considerations
    - Role of Epinephrine
    - Steroid Use and Delayed Reactions

Chapter 4: Overview of Shock

1. Definition
    - Pathophysiology of Shock
    - Classification of Shock Types

2. Stages of Shock
    - Preshock (Compensated)
    - Shock (Decompensated)
    - End Stage (Irreversible)

3. Vasopressors and Inotropes
    - Vasopressors: Noradrenaline, Adrenaline, Phenylephrine
    - Inotropes: Dopamine, Dobutamine

4. Management Principles
    - Hypovolemic Shock
    - Septic Shock
    - Cardiogenic Shock
    - Obstructive Shock
    - Neurogenic Shock
    - Adrenal Crisis

5. Key Considerations
    - Fluid Resuscitation Priorities

- Vasopressor Use in Hypovolemic Shock

Chapter 5: Septic Shock

1. Introduction
    - Sepsis and Systemic Inflammatory Response Syndrome (SIRS)
    - Sepsis-3 Definitions

2. qSOFA and SOFA Scoring Systems
    - qSOFA Criteria
    - SOFA Score for Organ Dysfunction

3. National Early Warning Score 2 (NEWS2)
    - Scoring System for Sepsis Detection

4. Management of Severe Sepsis and Septic Shock
    - Fluid Resuscitation
    - Antibiotic Therapy
    - Source Control
    - Temperature Management

5. Additional Measures

- Hyperglycemia Management
- Blood Transfusion Criteria
- Lactate Clearance Monitoring

Chapter 6: Airway Management in the Emergency Department

1. Introduction
   - Importance of Airway Management in the ED
   - Challenges and Preparation

2. Airway Assessment in Emergency Settings
   - MOANS: Assessing Difficult Mask Ventilation
   - LEMON: Assessing a Difficult Airway

3. Identification of a Compromised Airway
   - Clinical Signs of Airway Compromise
   - Scenarios Associated with a Difficult Airway

4. Preparation for Endotracheal Intubation
   - Optimal Positioning

- Essential Equipment and Medication
- Team Communication

5. Alignment of Airway Axes
    - Importance of Aligning Airway Axes for Successful Intubation
    - Special Considerations (e.g., Cervical Spine Stability, Obese Patients)

6. Laryngeal Visualization
    - Cormack and Lehane Grading
    - Evaluating Laryngeal View During Intubation

7. Laryngeal Mask Airway (LMA)
    - Indications and Size Selection
    - Proper Placement and Function

Chapter 7: Respiratory Support

1. Introduction
    - The Role of Oxygen Therapy in Respiratory Support

2. Oxygen Delivery Methods
   - Face Masks and FiO_2 Calculation
   - Flow Rate Adjustments by Device

3. Potential Risks of Oxygen Therapy
   - Physical, Functional, and Cytotoxic Risks

4. Types of Respiratory Failure
   - Type 1 (Oxygenation Failure)
   - Type 2 (Ventilatory Failure)

5. Ventilatory Support Modalities
   - Noninvasive Ventilation (NIV)
   - Types: NIPPV, CPAP, BiPAP
   - Indications and Contraindications
   - BiPAP Initial Settings

6. Invasive Ventilation
   - Indications for Intubation
   - Initial Ventilator Settings
   - Monitoring and Complications

Chapter 8: Fluid Therapy

1. Introduction
    - Body Water Distribution
    - Fluid Homeostasis

2. Choice of Intravenous Fluids
    - Normal Saline (0.9% NS)
    - Ringer Lactate (RL)
    - Dextrose Normal Saline (DNS)
    - 5% Dextrose
    - Hypotonic Saline Solutions (½ NS, ¼ NS)
    - Hypertonic Saline (3% NaCl)

3. Fluid Distribution and Effects
    - Effect on Intracellular and Extracellular Compartments

4. Crystalloid Composition
    - Composition of Common Crystalloids

Chapter 9: Sodium

1. Introduction
    - Importance of Sodium

2. Hyponatremia
    - Causes and Symptoms
    - Pseudohyponatremia
    - Management Guidelines

3. Hypernatremia
    - Causes and Symptoms
    - Management Strategies
    - Adrogue–Madias Formula

Chapter 10: Potassium

1. Introduction
    - Role in the Body

2. Hypokalemia
    - Causes, Symptoms, and ECG Changes
    - Management Strategies

3. Hyperkalemia
    - Causes and Symptoms
    - Treatment Strategies
    - Cardioprotection
    - Intracellular Shifting

- Potassium Excretion

Chapter 11: Calcium

1. Introduction
   - Forms of Calcium in Circulation

2. Hypocalcemia
   - Causes, Symptoms, and Management
   - Acute and Chronic Management

3. Hypercalcemia
   - Causes, Symptoms, and Management Strategies
   - Medications for Severe Hypercalcemia

Chapter 12: Magnesium

1. Introduction
   - Importance of Magnesium

2. Hypomagnesemia
   - Causes, Symptoms, and Treatment

3. Hypermagnesemia
    - Causes, Symptoms, and Management
    - Use of Calcium Gluconate and Dialysis

Chapter 13: Acid-Base Abnormalities

1. Introduction
    - Normal Reference Ranges
    - Compensatory Mechanisms in Acid-Base Disorders

2. Compensation Rules
    - Metabolic Disorders
    - Respiratory Disorders

3. Interpreting Arterial Blood Gas (ABG) Results
    - Detailed History and Primary Issue
    - Evaluating PaO2 and PaO2/FiO2 Ratio
    - pH and Base Excess (BE) Evaluation
    - Anion Gap Calculation
    - Electrolytes and Glucose Review
    - Lactate and Methemoglobin Analysis

4. Comparison of ABG and Venous Blood Gas (VBG) Analysis
   - pH, Lactate, HCO3, PaCO2, PaO2

5. Clinical Utility of ABG and VBG
   - ABG vs. VBG in Clinical Practice
   - Indications for VBG
   - Indications for ABG

6. Summary
   - When to Use ABG and VBG
   - Clinical Integration for Optimal Management

Chapter 14: Antibiotic Protocol for Common Conditions

1. Introduction

2. Acute Gastroenteritis

3. Bacillary Dysentery

4. Giardiasis

5. Typhoid Fever

6. Cholangitis and Acute Cholecystitis

7. Cellulitis

8. Necrotizing Fasciitis

9. Septic Arthritis

10. Acute Meningitis

11. Dengue Fever

Chapter 15: Dengue

1. Introduction

2. Clinical Presentation and Case Definitions
    - Dengue Fever
    - Dengue Hemorrhagic Fever (DHF)
    - Dengue Shock Syndrome (DSS)

3. Management Strategies
   - Supportive Care
   - Monitoring
   - Treatment

Chapter 16: Malaria

1. Introduction

2. Clinical Presentation

3. Diagnosis

4. Treatment
   - First-line Treatment
   - Severe Malaria

Chapter 17: Tuberculosis

1. Introduction

2. Clinical Presentation

3. Diagnosis

4. Treatment
   - First-line Drugs
   - Drug-Resistant TB

Chapter 18: Sepsis

1. Introduction

2. Pathophysiology

3. Clinical Presentation

4. Diagnosis

5. Management
   - Early Goal-Directed Therapy
   - Antibiotic Therapy
   - Supportive Care

Chapter 19: Influenza and H1N1

1. Introduction

2. Clinical Features

3. Investigations

4. High-Risk Groups

5. Management
    - Low-risk Management
    - High-risk Management

6. Post-Exposure Prophylaxis

7. Vaccination

Chapter 20: COVID-19

1. Introduction

2. Clinical Presentation

3. Diagnostic Evaluation

4. Management by Severity

- Mild Cases
- Moderate Cases
- Severe Cases

5. Prevention and Control

Chapter 21: Vaccination Strategies for Emerging Respiratory Viruses

1. Introduction

2. Influenza Vaccination

3. COVID-19 Vaccination

4. Challenges in Vaccination Efforts

5. Future Directions

Chapter 22: Food Poisoning and Acute Gastroenteritis

1. Introduction

2. Non-inflammatory Diarrhea
   - Clinical Features

3. Inflammatory Diarrhea
   - Clinical Features

4. Management
   - Hydration Therapy
   - Symptomatic Management
   - Antibiotic Use
   - Precautions

5. Etiology Based on Incubation Period
   - Very Short Incubation Period (1–6 Hours)
   - Short Incubation Period (10–48 Hours)
   - Long Incubation Period (1–5 Days)

Chapter 23: Urinary Tract Infections (UTI)

1. Introduction

2. Lower UTI (Cystitis)

3. Upper UTI (Pyelonephritis)

4. Management
    - Uncomplicated UTI
    - Complicated UTI
    - Asymptomatic Bacteriuria

5. Diagnostic Investigations
    - Urinalysis
    - Imaging

Chapter 24: Acute Central Nervous System (CNS) Infections

1. Introduction

2. Meningitis
    - Symptoms

3. Encephalitis
    - Symptoms

Chapter 25: Tetanus

1. Introduction

2. Severity Assessment Analysis
   - Patel and Joag Scoring System

3. Therapy
   - Immediate Treatment
   - Antibiotics

4. General Management
   - Airway Maintenance
   - Environmental Modifications
   - Sedation and Spasm Control
   - Nutritional and Hydration Support

5. Active Immunization

6. Tetanus Prophylaxis Protocol Analysis
   - Clean or Minor Wounds
   - Contaminated or Severe Wounds
   - Timing Considerations

Chapter 26: Antibiotic Doses and Spectrum

1. Introduction

- Importance of Accurate Antibiotic Selection
- Role of Empiric Therapy

2. Antibiotic Doses and Their Spectrum
    - Crystalline Penicillin
    - Coverage: Gram-positive organisms, Neisseria , Anaerobes
    - Amoxicillin and Ampicillin
    - Coverage: Gram-positive organisms, Fusobacterium
    - Cloxacillin
    - Coverage: Methicillin-sensitive Staphylococcus aureus, Anaerobes
    - Piperacillin–Tazobactam and Cefoperazone–Sulbactam
    - Coverage: Multidrug-resistant gram-negative pathogens, Pseudomonas aeruginosa
    - First-Generation Cephalosporins (Cefazolin, Cephalexin)
    - Coverage: Gram-positive organisms, Limited gram-negative bacteria (E. coli, Klebsiella)

- Second-Generation Cephalosporins (Cefuroxime)
- Coverage: Expanded gram-negative spectrum
- Third-Generation Cephalosporins (Ceftriaxone, Ceftazidime)
- Coverage: Resistant gram-negative pathogens
- Vancomycin and Linezolid
- Coverage: Methicillin-resistant Staphylococcus aureus (MRSA), Resistant enterococci
- Special Considerations: Oral option for outpatient treatment with Linezolid
- Fluoroquinolones (Ciprofloxacin, Levofloxacin)
- Coverage: Gram-negative pathogens, Atypical bacteria (Legionella, Chlamydia)
- Macrolides (Azithromycin)
- Coverage: Atypical infections, Gram-negative organisms
- Tetracyclines (Doxycycline)

- Coverage: Atypical infections, Intracellular pathogens (Rickettsia, Mycoplasma pneumoniae)

3. Conclusion
    - Key Takeaways: Importance of proper dosing and spectrum in antibiotic selection
    - Impact on Empiric Therapy and Patient Outcomes

Chapter 27: General Measures

1. Introduction
    - Importance of comprehensive history and reliable information
    - Role of decontamination methods

2. Gastric Lavage
    - Indications and contraindications
    - Technique and procedure

3. Activated Charcoal
    - Indications and dosage

- Multidose activated charcoal
- Contraindications

Chapter 28: Drug Overdose

1. Introduction
   - Overview of drug overdose causes and challenges in clinical management

2. General Management of Drug Overdose
   - Stabilization, IV access, diagnostic evaluation, decontamination, and antidote administration

3. Specific Overdoses and Their Management
   - Acetaminophen Overdose
   - Symptoms, toxic dose, and management with N-acetylcysteine (NAC)
   - Tricyclic Antidepressant (TCA) Overdose
   - Symptoms, management with sodium bicarbonate, glucagon, and more
   - Other Overdoses
   - Benzodiazepines, Beta-blockers, Calcium Channel Blockers

Chapter 29: Insecticide Poisoning

1. Organophosphorus Compounds
   - Types, clinical features, neurological and cardiovascular manifestations
   - Diagnosis and management strategies

2. Organochlorine Compounds
   - Clinical presentation and management

3. Carbamates
   - Clinical features and management

4. Pyrethroids
   - Types and management

5. Paraquat Poisoning
   - Clinical presentation and management strategies

Chapter 30: Rodenticides

1. Introduction

- Use and toxicity of rodenticides, with a focus on India

2. Types of Rodenticides
   - Anticoagulants, Inorganic Rodenticides, Other Rodenticides

3. Anticoagulants
   - Treatment protocols for bleeding and prolonged INR

4. Phosphorus-Based Compounds
   - Aluminum and Zinc Phosphides: Clinical features and management

Chapter 31: Plant Poisons

1. Oleander (Nerium oleander) and Yellow Oleander (Thevetia)
   - Toxic Components
   - Clinical Presentation
   - Management
   - Early Intervention
   - Cardiac Management

- Hyperkalemia Treatment
- Hypokalemia Management
- Antidote

2. Oduvanthalai (Cleistanthus collinus)
    - Toxic Components
    - Clinical Presentation
    - Management
    - Early Intervention
    - Electrolyte Imbalance Correction
    - Cardiac Monitoring

3. Datura (Datura stramonium)
    - Toxic Components
    - Clinical Presentation
    - Management
    - Supportive Care
    - Monitoring for Cholinergic Crisis

4. Strychnine (Strychnos nux-vomica)
    - Toxic Components
    - Clinical Presentation
    - Management
    - Muscle Relaxation

- Airway Management
- IV Fluids
- No Role for Gastric Lavage

5. Conclusion
    - Systematic Approach to Plant Poisoning Management

Chapter 32: Snake Bites

1. Introduction
    - Overview of Venomous Snakes in India
    - The "Big Four" Snakes
    - Other Venomous Snakes

2. First Aid
    - Tourniquet Application
    - Limb Immobilization
    - Avoid Cooling and Incision

3. Examination and Investigations
    - Identifying Fang Marks
    - Neurotoxicity Symptoms
    - Hemotoxicity Symptoms

- Coagulation Status
- Other Investigations

4. Management
    - Pain Relief
    - Antibiotics
    - Tetanus Prophylaxis

5. Anti Snake Venom (ASV)
    - Types and Effectiveness
    - Dry Bites and ASV Administration
    - Premedication
    - Dosage and Administration

6. Management of Anaphylaxis
    - Immediate Steps
    - Restarting ASV Infusion

7. Additional Management Considerations
    - Respiratory Failure
    - Bleeding Management
    - Shock Management
    - Renal Failure
    - Ptosis Management

8. Cost and Regional Variations
   - Cost of ASV
   - Regional Variations in Venom Efficacy

9. Conclusion
   - Snake Bite Management Overview

Chapter 33: Insect Envenomation

1. Scorpion Stings
   - Clinical Features
   - Investigations
   - Management
   - First Aid
   - Pain Relief
   - Vaccination
   - Antibiotics
   - Prazosin and Other Treatments

2. Centipede Bites
   - Clinical Features
   - Management

3. Bee and Wasp Stings (Hymenoptera Species)
    - Local Reactions and Management
    - Anaphylaxis
    - Stinger Removal and Wound Care

4. Other Insect Bites
    - Beetles, Caterpillars, and Millipedes
    - Spider Bites

Chapter 34: Substance Abuse

1. Opioids
    - Signs and Symptoms of Overdose
    - Management and Naloxone Dosing Guidelines

2. Cannabis (Marijuana)
    - Signs of Intoxication
    - Management of Acute Intoxication
    - Cannabis Hyperemesis Syndrome

3. Amphetamines
    - Acute Intoxication Management
    - Hypertension and Seizures

4. Cocaine
    - Symptoms and Complications
    - Acute Intoxication Management

5. Ecstasy (MDMA)
    - Complications
    - Management

6. Lysergic Acid Diethylamide (LSD)
    - Symptoms and Management

7. Summary
    - Overview of Substance Abuse Management

Chapter 35: Miscellaneous Toxicological Emergencies

1. Corrosive Poisoning
    - Types of Corrosive Agents
    - Acids vs. Alkalis
    - Common Corrosives
    - Investigations

2. Management Guidelines
   - Acute Ingestion (Within 24 Hours)
   - Initial Management
   - Endoscopy and Follow-Up
   - Chronic Ingestion (After 24 Hours)
   - Surgical Interventions and Follow-Up

List of Abbreviations

ECG – Electrocardiogram

EKG – Electrocardiograph

ACS – Acute Coronary Syndrome

ATDs – Antithyroid Drugs

RAI – Radioactive Iodine

PPT – Postpartum Thyroiditis

CT – Computed Tomography

MRI – Magnetic Resonance Imaging

FNAB – Fine Needle Aspiration Biopsy

TSH – Thyroid Stimulating Hormone

T3 – Triiodothyronine

T4 – Thyroxine

TSI – Thyroid Stimulating Immunoglobulins

DCT – Doppler Cardiac Testing

PET – Positron Emission Tomography

CVD – Cardiovascular Disease

AHA – American Heart Association

HRT – Hormone Replacement Therapy

IUGR – Intrauterine Growth Restriction

PIH – Pregnancy-Induced Hypertension

DVT – Deep Vein Thrombosis

TIA – Transient Ischemic Attack

PE – Pulmonary Embolism

VSD – Ventricular Septal Defect

PVD – Peripheral Vascular Disease

IVF – In Vitro Fertilization

OB/GYN – Obstetrics and Gynecology

LDL – Low-Density Lipoprotein

HDL – High-Density Lipoprotein

CABG – Coronary Artery Bypass Grafting

ICU – Intensive Care Unit

ICD – Implantable Cardioverter Defibrillator

PPI – Proton Pump Inhibitor

NSAIDs – Nonsteroidal Anti-inflammatory Drugs

COPD – Chronic Obstructive Pulmonary Disease

ICU – Intensive Care Unit

RA – Rheumatoid Arthritis

FNAC – Fine Needle Aspiration Cytology

CTO – Chronic Total Occlusion

HF – Heart Failure

CHF – Congestive Heart Failure

EEG – Electroencephalogram

CVS – Cardiovascular System

NGT – Nasogastric Tube

IV – Intravenous

PRBC – Packed Red Blood Cells

CABG – Coronary Artery Bypass Grafting

SLE – Systemic Lupus Erythematosus

ASHD – Atherosclerotic Heart Disease

PRA – Panel Reactive Antibody

CK-MB – Creatine Kinase-MB

TNT – Troponin T

PFT – Pulmonary Function Test

O2 – Oxygen

SCT – Stem Cell Therapy

RAI – Radioactive Iodine

TBG – Thyroxine Binding Globulin

Section 1: Basic Life Support and Management of Cardiac Arrest

Chapter 1:
Basic Life Support (BLS

Introduction

Basic Life Support (BLS) is a critical initial intervention provided to individuals facing life-threatening emergencies, such as cardiac arrest or severe injuries, until advanced medical care becomes available. This vital care can be performed by healthcare professionals like doctors, nurses, paramedics, or even trained bystanders.

The primary objective of BLS is the rapid restoration of cerebral perfusion to minimize brain damage, as the brain is highly sensitive to inadequate blood flow.

The American Heart Association (AHA) periodically updates its BLS and Advanced Cardiac Life Support (ACLS) guidelines. The latest 2020 AHA guidelines emphasize the following:

Following the sequence of Circulation–Airway–Breathing (C–A–B).

Ensuring high-quality cardiopulmonary resuscitation (CPR).

Administering naloxone for suspected opioid overdoses.

Using a defibrillator promptly in cases of witnessed cardiac arrest.

Administering epinephrine as early as possible.

Monitoring arterial waveform using ETCO2.

Utilizing real-time audio-visual feedback to enhance team performance.

Key Components of Basic Life Support (BLS)

BLS involves four essential steps:

1. Chest Compressions

2. Airway Management

3. Breathing Support

4. Defibrillation

Overview of BLS Steps

1. Scene Safety and Initial Assessment

Ensure the environment is safe for both the rescuer and the victim.

Relocate the victim from hazardous areas to a safe location.

2. Recognition of Cardiac Arrest

Check the victim's responsiveness by tapping their shoulder and asking, "Are you all right?"

Assess for normal breathing patterns. If the victim is unresponsive and not breathing or only gasping, call for help.

Check for a carotid pulse within 5–10 seconds. If no pulse is felt, initiate the emergency response system.

3. Activating the Emergency Response System

If alone without a mobile phone, first activate the emergency response system and retrieve an AED before starting CPR.

If assistance is available, delegate tasks to retrieve the AED and begin CPR immediately.

4. Starting CPR

Chest Compressions: Position the victim on a firm surface in a supine position. Place the heel of one hand on the lower half of the sternum, interlock fingers, and keep arms straight. Push hard and fast, allowing for full chest recoil while minimizing interruptions.

Rescue Breaths: Open the airway using the head tilt-chin lift method unless a spinal injury is suspected, in which case use the jaw thrust technique. Provide two breaths after every 30 compressions using a mask device if available, and observe for visible chest rise.

5. Automated External Defibrillator (AED)

Once the AED is available, follow its prompts. Continue CPR cycles (30 compressions: 2 breaths) until the device is ready to analyze the rhythm and deliver a shock if indicated.

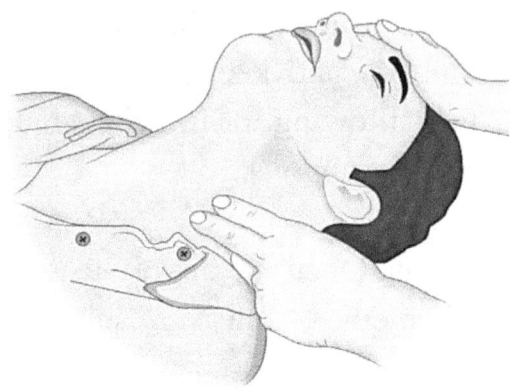

Figure 1-1: Carotid pulse check.

Chest Compressions

High-quality cardiopulmonary resuscitation (CPR) is essential to improving survival rates in cardiac arrest cases. Providers performing Basic Life Support (BLS) should adhere to the following key principles to ensure effective chest compressions:

Prompt Initiation: Begin chest compressions within 10 seconds of identifying cardiac arrest.

Rate and Depth: Maintain a compression rate of 100–120 per minute. Compress the chest to the appropriate depth:

Adults: At least 5 cm (2 inches).

Children: Approximately 5 cm (2 inches).

Infants: Approximately 4 cm (1½ inches).

Complete Recoil: Allow the chest to fully recoil after each compression to maximize cardiac output.

Minimize Interruptions: Limit pauses in compressions to less than 10 seconds.

Compression-Only CPR: For a lay rescuer or single rescuer, compression-only CPR is sufficient until additional help or equipment becomes available.

Effective Ventilations: Provide rescue breaths that visibly lift the chest. If an advanced airway is in place, administer one breath every 6 seconds (10 breaths per minute).

Airway Management

In unconscious individuals, the airway may become obstructed due to relaxation of the tongue and pharyngeal muscles. To ensure proper airflow and enable rescue breaths, BLS providers can use the following techniques:

Methods to Open the Airway:

1. Head Tilt-Chin Lift: This is the preferred method in patients without suspected head or spinal injuries.

Place one hand on the victim's forehead and apply gentle backward pressure.

Use the fingers of the other hand to lift the chin forward.

2. Jaw Thrust: This technique is used when a head or cervical spine injury is suspected.

Place your fingers behind the angles of the lower jaw.

Push the jaw upward without tilting the head backward.

Note: Avoid using the head tilt-chin lift maneuver in suspected spinal injuries to prevent further harm.

Evidence-Based Practices

Studies consistently demonstrate that timely and uninterrupted chest compressions combined with effective airway management significantly enhance outcomes in cardiac arrest patients. CPR guidelines emphasize a compression-first approach, especially for bystanders, to address the critical need for circulation. Additionally, airway techniques tailored to the clinical context can optimize oxygen delivery while minimizing the risk of complications.

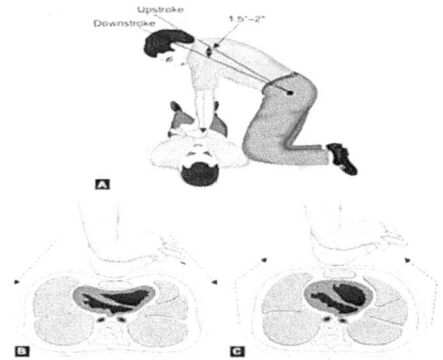

Figure 1-2A to C: Technique of chest compression

Methods for Opening the Airway

Ensuring an open airway is crucial in unresponsive patients to facilitate effective ventilation and oxygen delivery. Two primary techniques are used, depending on the patient's condition and the presence of suspected cervical spine injury:

1. Head Tilt–Chin Lift

This maneuver is the preferred method for opening the airway in patients without suspected cervical spine injuries. It works by lifting the tongue off the posterior pharynx to clear the airway.

Steps:

Place one hand on the patient's forehead and gently tilt the head backward by applying downward pressure.

With the other hand, position the tips of your index and middle fingers under the chin (mentum of the mandible) and lift the chin upward.

Key Consideration:

Avoid this technique if a cervical spine injury is suspected, as it may exacerbate spinal damage.

2. Jaw Thrust

The jaw thrust technique is specifically indicated for patients with suspected head or neck injuries. This approach minimizes neck movement while effectively displacing the mandible to prevent airway obstruction caused by the tongue.

Steps:

Position yourself at the patient's head, with one hand on each side of the head. Rest your elbows on the surface supporting the patient.

Place your fingers under the angles of the mandible.

Lift the jaw upward and forward using both hands, displacing the jaw and tongue anteriorly.

Key Mechanism:

By moving the jaw forward, this method prevents the tongue from collapsing into the airway, ensuring it remains patentable without compromising the cervical spine.

Evidence-Based Insights

Research highlights that the head tilt–chin lift method effectively clears the airway in most patients without spinal trauma. Conversely, the jaw thrust is recommended in trauma settings to protect the cervical spine. Proper application of these techniques, tailored to the patient's condition, is critical for optimal airway management and improved outcomes.

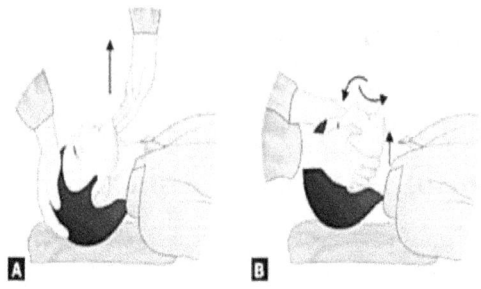

Figure 3A & B: (A) Head tilt–chin lift; and (B) Jaw thrust.

Precautions During Airway Management

To ensure effective airway management and ventilation, it is essential to avoid errors that may obstruct the airway or reduce the effectiveness of interventions:

Caution

Avoid pressing deeply under the chin: Excessive pressure on the soft tissue beneath the chin may inadvertently block the airway.

Do not use the thumb to lift the chin: This approach is less effective and may cause unintended issues.

Keep the victim's mouth slightly open: Closing the mouth completely can obstruct airflow, impeding proper ventilation.

Ventilation and Respiratory Arrest Management

Respiratory arrest occurs when the patient's breathing is inadequate to sustain oxygenation or completely absent. Addressing respiratory arrest requires prompt and systematic intervention to prevent hypoxia and further complications.

Key Components of Management

1. Administer supplemental oxygen: Helps maintain adequate oxygenation.

2. Ensure airway patency: Use basic airway techniques or adjuncts to keep the airway open.

3. Suction as needed: Clear any secretions or debris obstructing the airway.

4. Provide basic ventilation: Use a bag-mask device to deliver effective ventilation.

5. Secure an advanced airway: If indicated, intubation or other advanced methods may be necessary.

6. Identify and address underlying causes: Consider reversible factors contributing to respiratory arrest.

Basic Airway Adjuncts

In unresponsive patients, loss of throat muscle tone may cause the tongue to obstruct the airway. While manual techniques like the head tilt–chin lift or jaw thrust are essential, adjuncts like the oropharyngeal airway (OPA) and nasopharyngeal airway (NPA) can enhance ventilation during resuscitation.

Oropharyngeal Airway (OPA)

Indications: Used exclusively in unconscious patients to prevent the tongue from blocking the airway.

Choosing the Correct Size:

Measure the distance between the first incisor and the angle of the mandible.

Selecting an OPA that is too large can obstruct the glottis, causing airway blockage.

Technique: Insert with care to avoid trauma to the oral cavity.

Nasopharyngeal Airway (NPA)

Usage: May be employed in semi-conscious patients where the OPA is contraindicated.

Selection: Ensure proper sizing to avoid nasal trauma.

Evidence-Based Practice

Studies highlight that inappropriate sizing or improper insertion of airway adjuncts can lead to complications such as oral trauma, airway obstruction, or ineffective ventilation. Adequate training and adherence to protocols significantly improve outcomes in respiratory arrest management.

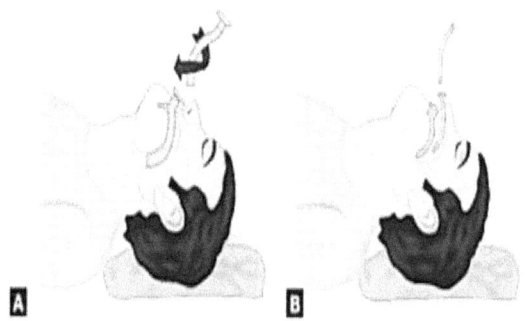

Figure 1-4A & B: Overview of basic airway adjuncts: demonstrating the placement and function of the oropharyngeal airway (OPA) and nasopharyngeal airway (NPA).

Nasopharyngeal Airway Insertion Guidelines:

Adults: Insert the tube with the concave side facing upward and rotate it 180 degrees once it reaches the back of the throat.

Children and Infants: Insert the tube with the concave side downward, using a tongue depressor to hold the tongue forward.

Contraindications: Avoid use in conscious patients, as it may induce a gag reflex, potentially causing vomiting.

Nasopharyngeal Airway Insertion:

Size Selection: Choose a size based on the distance from the tip of the nose to the earlobe.

Insertion: Lubricate the tube with anesthetic jelly and insert it through one nostril, ensuring the flared end rests at the nostril.

Indication: Suitable for semi-conscious patients.

Contraindications: Should not be used in patients with skull base fractures or nasal bleeding.

Rescue Breaths Guidelines:

Rescue breaths can be administered via mouth-to-mouth or mouth-to-nose. A mask or improvised device (such as a rolled board) may also be used.

Provide two rescue breaths after every 30 chest compressions.

Each rescue breath should be delivered sharply and last no longer than 1 second.

Ensure adequate tidal volume for visible chest rise, but avoid over-inflating the lungs.

Bag-Mask Ventilation (BMV):

BMV Device: A self-inflating reservoir bag, mask, one-way valve (prevents rebreathing of exhaled air), and an oxygen port for supplemental oxygen.

E–C Clamp Technique: This technique ensures effective bag-mask ventilation and can be performed by one or two rescuers.

E–C Clamp Technique

Single Rescuer: Form a "C" with the thumb and first finger around the mask and use the remaining fingers to lift the jaw (forming an "E") while the other hand squeezes the bag to ventilate the patient.

Two Rescuers: One rescuer holds the mask with both hands using the E–C technique, while the other squeezes the bag to provide ventilation for 1 second.

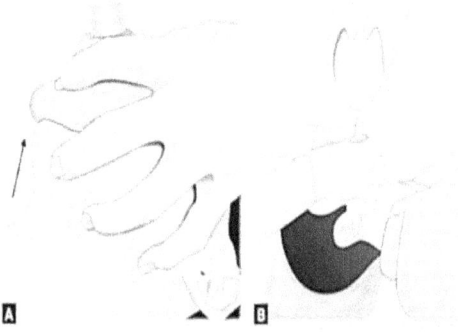

Figure 1-5A & B: E–C clamp technique: Single rescuer and double rescuer.

Steps for Bag-Mask Ventilation

1. Position the Mask: Place the mask over the victim's face, ensuring it covers the nose and mouth, with the nasal end aligned with the bridge of the nose, and not extending over the

eyes. The mask's bottom should rest just under the chin.

2. Airway Adjunct: If available, use an airway adjunct to assist in keeping the airway open.

3. Secure the Mask: Hold the mask using the E–C technique with one hand, or use both hands if a second rescuer is present.

4. Apply Pressure: Ensure firm pressure is applied to create a good seal between the mask and the face.

5. Ventilation: Squeeze the bag steadily, delivering enough air to make the chest rise. Use a tidal volume of approximately 8–10 mL/kg.

6. Avoid Explosive Squeezing: Squeeze the bag slowly over about one second, avoiding rapid or forceful compression.

7. Oxygen Supply: If available, connect the bag-mask device to a reservoir bag with supplemental oxygen.

8. Ventilation Frequency: Administer two ventilations after every 30 chest compressions for patients without an advanced airway.

9. Asynchronous Ventilation: For patients with an advanced airway, provide ventilation every 8–10 seconds (6–8 breaths per minute).

Basic Life Support/CPR for Children (Ages 1 Year to Puberty)

The child CPR sequence is similar to adult CPR but with key differences:

Compression-Ventilation Ratio:

Two-rescuer CPR: 15:2

Lone rescuer CPR: 30:2

Compression Depth: Compress at least one-third of the chest depth (approximately 5 cm or 2 inches).

Compression Technique: Use either one or two-handed chest compressions, depending on the child's size.

Defibrillation Dosage:

First shock: 2 J/kg

Second shock: 4 J/kg

Subsequent shocks: >4 J/kg

Maximum dose: 10 J/kg or the adult dose

Activation of Emergency Response System:

In cases of unwitnessed arrest, perform 2 minutes of CPR before activating the emergency system and retrieving a defibrillator.

If witnessed arrest, immediately activate the emergency system and retrieve the defibrillator.

Basic Life Support/CPR for Infants

Key differences for infant CPR:

Pulse Check: Use the brachial artery to check the pulse in infants.

Chest Compression Technique:

Single rescuer: Use the two-finger technique.

Two rescuers: Use the two-thumb encircling technique (Fig. 6).

Compression Depth: Compress at least one-third of the chest depth (approximately 4 cm or 1½ inches).

Compression-Ventilation Ratio:

Two-rescuer CPR: 15:2

Lone rescuer CPR: 30:2

Defibrillation Dosage:

First shock: 2 J/kg

Second shock: 4 J/kg

Subsequent shocks: >4 J/kg

Maximum dose: 10 J/kg

Activation of the emergency response system is done similarly to the procedure for children.

Defibrillation and Cardioversion

Defibrillation: This is the delivery of a shock that is not synchronized with the cardiac cycle. The shock depolarizes all the cardiac tissue, rendering it refractory and preventing the continuation of the abnormal electrical circuit. It is typically used in patients experiencing pulseless cardiac arrest.

Cardioversion: Unlike defibrillation, cardioversion delivers a shock synchronized with the QRS complex, targeting only the active arrhythmic circuit. It is used to correct arrhythmias in awake patients.

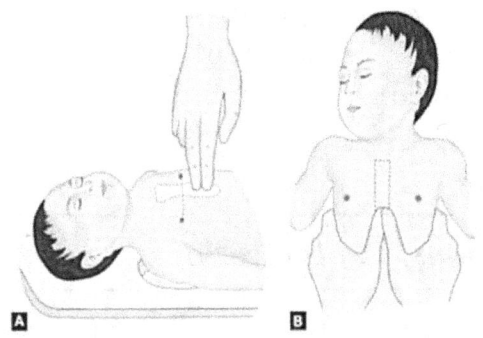

Figure 1-6A & B: Technique of chest compression in children.

Key Differences Between Cardioversion and Defibrillation

Cardioversion	Fibrillation
Procedure Type: elective	**Procedure Type:** emergency
Patient Status: Patient is often away, sedated	**Patient Status:** Patient is unconscious
Shock	**Shock**

Synchronization: Shock is synchronized with the QRS Complex	Synchronization: Shock is unsynchronized
Indications	**Indications**
Unstable Atrial fibrillation /flutter	Pulseless Ventricular Tachycardia
Refractory supraventricular Tachycardia	Ventricular fibrillation
Unstable ventricular tachycardia with pulse	
Energy Level	**Energy Level**
50 - 200j (biphasic)	200j (biphasic)
360j (monophasic)	360j (monophasic)

Monophasic vs. Biphasic Defibrillators

Monophasic Defibrillators: These defibrillators deliver a shock in one direction, from one electrode to another. They require higher energy (typically 360 J) and have various drawbacks, such as causing more damage to the heart tissue. As a result, they are rarely used in modern emergency care settings.

Biphasic Defibrillators: These devices are more efficient and cause less cardiac damage by delivering a shock in two phases: the first half of the waveform goes in one direction, and the second half is reversed. Biphasic defibrillators typically use lower energy levels and are preferred for defibrillation today, including in automated external defibrillators (AEDs), manual defibrillators, and implantable defibrillators.

Using an Automatic External Defibrillator (AED)

1. Read Instructions: Follow the AED's provided instructions.

2. Place Pads: Attach the pads to the chest, with the right pad below the right clavicle and the left pad positioned on the left inferior-lateral chest wall.

3. Alternate Placement: For patients with a thoracic injury, the pads can be placed in the axillary regions (right and left).

4. Turn On AED: Power up the AED and follow the voice instructions.

5. Rhythm Analysis: The AED will automatically analyze the heart rhythm and will deliver a shock if a shockable rhythm is detected.

Using a Biphasic Defibrillator

1. Power On: Turn the defibrillator to manual mode.

2. Set Energy: Select the appropriate energy dose (e.g., 200 J for adults and 2 J/kg for children).

3. Prepare Paddles: Apply gel to the paddles, and place them on the chest (sternal paddle below the right clavicle, apex paddle on the left lateral chest).

4. Safety: Ensure the resuscitation team stays clear, and disconnect the oxygen circuit.

5. Shock Delivery: Press the discharge button on the paddles or the device to deliver the shock.

6. Resume CPR: Immediately restart CPR. Do not pause to check the pulse or rhythm post-shock.

Cardioversion Using a Biphasic Defibrillator

1. Patient Consent and Sedation: Obtain consent from the patient and administer appropriate sedation (e.g., ketamine 1 mg/kg or midazolam 2 mg plus fentanyl 50 μg).

2. Set Defibrillator: Power the defibrillator to manual mode, and select the energy dose (typically 50–200 J).

3. Prepare Paddles: Apply gel to the paddles or use pads, if available. Position the paddles as before (ternal below the right clavicle and apex on the left lateral chest).

4. Synchronize Shock: Set the defibrillator to synchronized mode.

5. Shock Delivery: Hold the paddles in place for at least 5 seconds while delivering the shock. Ensure the oxygen circuit is disconnected and the team stays clear.

6. Post-Shock Assessment: Check the pulse and rhythm immediately after the shock. If arrhythmia persists, administer another cardioversion with a higher energy dose.

Chapter 2
Management of Cardiac Arrest

Introduction

The successful revival of a cardiac arrest victim typically requires advanced technology and medical equipment, including defibrillators, intubation tools, oxygen, and medications. These interventions are most effectively administered in an emergency department (ED) where a skilled team—including doctors, nurses, and paramedics—works in coordination. The team leader is responsible for guiding the resuscitation efforts, delegating tasks, making treatment decisions, and providing constructive feedback to the team.

Upon identifying a cardiac arrest, it is essential to activate the emergency response system and follow the Basic Life Support (BLS) protocol.

This process generally includes the following steps:

1. Monitor the Cardiac Rhythm: The patient should be connected to a cardiac monitor to assess the rhythm and determine the appropriate actions.

2. Establish Venous Access: Start with establishing peripheral venous access. If two attempts fail, an intraosseous (IO) line should be used. In cases where intubation has already been performed, medications can be delivered via the endotracheal (ET) tube.

3. Maintain Airway Patency: If the patient is not intubated, insert an oropharyngeal or nasopharyngeal airway to keep the airway open and prevent the tongue from obstructing the airway until intubation can be completed.

4. Consider Reversible Causes: It is important to assess the potential reversible causes of cardiac arrest, often referred to as the "5Hs and 5Ts."

These include conditions like hypoxia, hypovolemia, and cardiac tamponade.

The following section outlines the drugs commonly used during cardiac arrest and those that can be administered through the ET tube.

Bradyarrhythmias

Bradyarrhythmias are characterized by a slow heart rate, typically below 60 beats per minute. This can include conditions such as third-degree atrioventricular (AV) block or sinus bradycardia. Treatment is necessary when bradycardia leads to inadequate blood flow to vital organs. This is usually observed when the heart rate falls below 50 beats per minute. Symptoms of unstable bradyarrhythmia can include:

Low blood pressure or signs of shock

Altered mental status

In these situations, it is critical to identify and address reversible causes, which can range from hypoxia and electrolyte imbalances to conditions like tension pneumothorax or cardiac tamponade.

Common Drugs in Cardiac Arrest

Several medications are commonly used during cardiac arrest, depending on the rhythm and underlying cause. These include:

Adrenaline (Epinephrine): Used in conditions such as ventricular fibrillation (VF), pulseless ventricular tachycardia (VT), pulseless electrical activity (PEA), and asystole. It is typically administered intravenously (IV) or intraosseously (IO), with doses repeated every 3 to 5 minutes.

Amiodarone: This drug is employed for refractory VF and VT. If the initial dose is ineffective, a second dose can be given.

Lidocaine: Often used for refractory VF and VT or stable VT, with the initial dose administered IV/IO, followed by a second dose if needed.

Atropine: This is the primary medication used for symptomatic bradycardia, particularly when the heart rate is extremely slow, often below 50 beats per minute. It is administered IV, with the dose repeated every 3 to 5 minutes up to a maximum amount.

Dopamine: This medication is used when bradycardia does not respond to atropine, or when there are signs of shock or low blood pressure despite the bradycardia. It is given as an infusion.

Magnesium sulfate: This drug is used to treat torsades de pointes, a type of abnormal heart rhythm associated with prolonged QT intervals.

In situations where intravenous (IV) or intraosseous (IO) access is difficult, some medications can be administered via the ET tube. When given through this route, the required dose is typically 2 to 3 times the standard IV dose.

Bradycardia Rhythms

Bradycardia refers to heart rhythms with a rate slower than 60 beats per minute. Various forms of bradycardia include:

Sinus Bradycardia: A regular rhythm with a consistent P-wave before each QRS complex.

First-degree AV Block: A regular rhythm, but the P-R interval is prolonged beyond 0.20 seconds.

Second-degree AV Block (Type 1 - Wenckebach): An irregular rhythm with progressively longer P-R intervals until a QRS complex is dropped.

Second-degree AV Block (Type 2): An irregular rhythm with a constant P-R interval, but with intermittent dropped QRS complexes.

Third-degree AV Block (Complete Heart Block): The P-wave and QRS complex are not related, and the rhythm is regular but independent between the atria and ventricles.

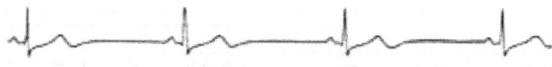

Figure 2-1: Sinus bradycardia.

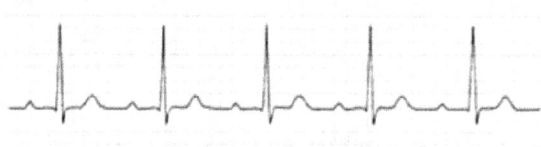

Figure 2-2: First-degree AV block.

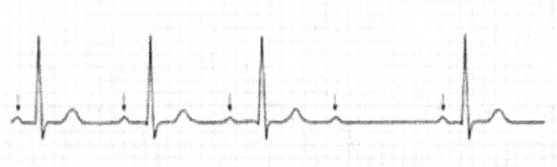

Figure 2-3: Second-degree Mobitz type 1 AV block (Wenckebach).

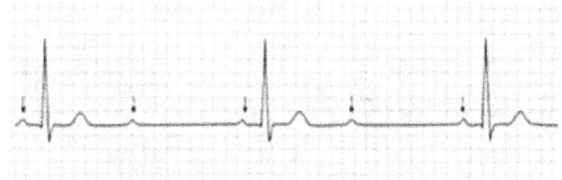

Figure 2-4: Second-degree Mobitz type 2 AV block.

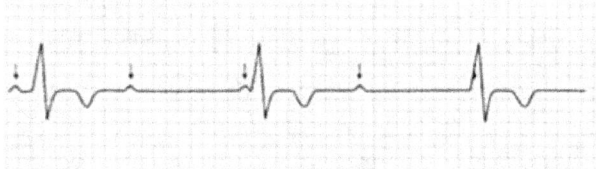

Figure 2-5: Third-degree AV block (complete heart block).

Management of Bradyarrhythmias

For patients with symptomatic bradycardia, the immediate administration of 1 mg of intravenous (IV) atropine is recommended as the first-line treatment. If this initial treatment is ineffective, other therapeutic options include:

Chronotropic agents: Administration of agents like adrenaline or dopamine via infusion.

Transcutaneous pacing: This technique provides an immediate solution by stimulating the heart externally.

Transvenous pacing: A more invasive procedure, used when other methods fail.

Reversible Causes of Bradycardia
In cases of symptomatic bradycardia, it is essential to identify and address potential reversible causes, including:

Hypoxia

Electrolyte imbalances such as hypokalemia or hyperkalemia

Organ-related issues like pneumothorax or raised intracranial pressure

Persistent Bradycardia Management

If bradycardia persists despite atropine administration, a chronotropic agent infusion should be initiated. If necessary, preparations for transcutaneous pacing should be made. If these measures fail, transvenous pacing and expert consultation are required.

Limitations of Atropine

Atropine is ineffective for high-degree atrioventricular (AV) blocks, such as second-degree Mobitz type II and third-degree AV block. In these cases, it is essential to skip atropine administration and move directly to transcutaneous pacing and chronotropic infusion.

Transcutaneous Pacing

Transcutaneous pacing is a procedure where electrical impulses are delivered through the skin to stimulate heart depolarization and subsequent contraction. This method provides short-term stabilization while the underlying issue is addressed or a more permanent solution is found.

Procedure for Transcutaneous Pacing:

1. Electrode Placement: Place the pacing pads in an anterior-posterior or anterior-lateral configuration, ensuring that the heart is aligned with the electrical axis.

2. ECG Leads: Attach ECG leads to monitor the pacing rhythm.

3. Setting the Pacemaker: Set the pacemaker rate to 60-80 beats per minute and begin pacing at 10 milliamps. Gradually increase the current until a

capture is observed (evidenced by wide QRS complexes and broad T waves on the ECG or a palpable pulse).

4. Current Adjustment: Once pacing is achieved, adjust the current to 5-10 milliamps above the threshold to ensure stable capture.

5. Patient Comfort: Note that transcutaneous pacing can be uncomfortable, particularly if high milliamps are used. Sedation may be considered in such cases.

Success Indicators: The success of the pacing is indicated by improved cardiac output, including a palpable pulse, increased blood pressure, and improved sensorium.

Pad Rotation: To prevent skin burns and discomfort, it is advised to rotate the pads every 4 hours.

Tachyarrhythmias

Tachyarrhythmias are defined as abnormal heart rhythms with a ventricular rate exceeding 100 beats per minute. The key clinical task is to determine whether the tachyarrhythmia is causing instability, such as hypotension, altered consciousness, ischemic chest pain, or acute pulmonary edema.

Initial Management:

1. Identify the rhythm and assess for signs of instability.

2. If the patient is unstable, synchronized cardioversion is required.

3. If stable, appropriate medical therapy should be administered and the patient should be closely monitored. Reversible causes (such as the 5Hs and 5Ts) should also be investigated and treated

Immediate Post Cardiac Arrest Care for Adults

Post Cardiac arrest care is essential for improving survival rates and ensuring neurological recovery after the return of spontaneous circulation (ROSC). ROSC is confirmed when there is sustained cardiac activity with peripheral perfusion and significant respiratory effort, as indicated by a rise in end-tidal CO2 (ETCO2).

Key Objectives:

Control body temperature: Use therapeutic hypothermia to optimize survival and neurological outcomes.

Airway management: Secure an advanced airway early.

Identify and treat underlying conditions, such as acute coronary syndromes.

Optimize ventilation: Ensure mechanical ventilation is appropriately managed to minimize lung injury.

Support organ function: Prevent multiorgan failure.

Key Steps:

1. Confirm ROSC.

2. Ventilation and Oxygenation: Target an oxygen saturation of 92–98%, intubate if necessary, and monitor ET tube placement.

3. Treat Hypotension: Administer IV fluids and vasopressors if required, and aim to maintain systolic blood pressure (SBP) >90 mm Hg or mean arterial pressure (MAP) >65 mm Hg.

4. Evaluate Sensorium: If the patient remains unconscious, induce therapeutic hypothermia. If responsive, treat underlying ACS and prepare for advanced care.

Cardiac Arrest in Pregnancy

Cardiac arrest during pregnancy presents unique challenges due to the physiological and anatomical changes in the body. Resuscitation efforts should prioritize the mother, but fetal viability must also be considered.

Resuscitation Considerations:

1. Intravenous Access: Ensure access above the diaphragm to avoid compression of the inferior vena cava by the gravid uterus.

2. Positioning During CPR: Tilt the patient to the left and manually displace the uterus to reduce vena cava compression and increase venous return.

3. Airway Management: Secure the airway early to prevent aspiration, which is more likely due to changes in gastrointestinal motility.

4. Defibrillation: Standard defibrillation protocols apply, but fetal monitors should be removed before defibrillation.

Fetal Monitoring:

Tocodynamometry: Should be used to monitor the fetus for signs of distress, such as tachycardia, loss of variability, or late decelerations.

Perimortem Cesarean Delivery:

In cases of maternal death or persistent fetal distress, perform a perimortem cesarean delivery within 5 minutes to improve fetal survival and potentially benefit maternal recovery.

Causes of Maternal Arrest:

Include obstetric causes such as hemorrhage, preeclampsia, or amniotic fluid embolism, and non-obstetric causes like pulmonary embolism or myocardial infarction.

Pediatric Cardiac Arrest

Cardiac arrest in children usually results from respiratory failure or shock, rather than arrhythmias. During resuscitation, prioritize airway management, oxygenation, and ventilation.

Resuscitation Protocol:

1. C-A-B Sequence: Begin with chest compressions, followed by airway management and breathing.

2. Compression-Ventilation Ratio: Use 30:2 for single rescuers and 15:2 for multiple rescuers.

3. Defibrillation: Use appropriate paddle sizes, ensuring a gap of at least 3 cm between the paddles. Use larger adult paddles for children over 10 kg and smaller paddles for infants under 10 kg.

Monitoring and Post-Arrest Care:

ETCO2 Monitoring: Target ETCO2 levels of >10-15 mmHg to indicate effective compressions.

Defibrillation: Ensure the correct paddle size is used based on the child's weight.

This comprehensive approach to the management of arrhythmias, including bradycardias, tachycardias, and special cases such as pregnancy and pediatric arrest, ensures that appropriate interventions are made at each stage of care, improving survival outcomes.

Section 2: Anaphylaxis, Shock, and Airway Management

Chapter 3
Understanding and Managing Anaphylaxis

Introduction

Anaphylaxis is a critical hypersensitivity reaction that occurs suddenly and poses a significant risk of fatality. It is primarily mediated by immunoglobulin E (IgE) and can be life-threatening without prompt intervention. The diagnosis is based on clinical criteria, typically involving multiple organ systems, as outlined below:

Skin and integumentary system: Affects 90% of cases

Respiratory system: Involved in 70% of cases

Gastrointestinal system: Impacts 45% of cases

Cardiovascular system: Observed in 45% of cases

Diagnostic Criteria for Anaphylaxis

Anaphylaxis is highly likely when one of the following three criteria is met:

1. Criterion 1

Acute onset (minutes to hours) with skin or mucosal involvement (e.g., hives, flushing, swelling of lips/tongue)

Accompanied by respiratory symptoms (e.g., wheezing, stridor, hypoxemia) or reduced blood pressure with signs of organ dysfunction (e.g., collapse, syncope).

2. Criterion 2

Rapid onset after exposure to a probable allergen, involving two or more of the following:

Skin or mucosal involvement

Respiratory compromise

Hypotension or associated symptoms

Persistent gastrointestinal symptoms (e.g., abdominal cramps, vomiting).

3. Criterion 3

Hypotension following exposure to a known allergen, defined as:

Systolic blood pressure <90 mmHg or a >30% drop from baseline in adults.

Note: Certain medications, including β-blockers and ACE inhibitors, can exacerbate anaphylaxis and interfere with treatment response.

Management of Anaphylaxis

Prompt and systematic management is essential to mitigate the risks associated with anaphylaxis. The following steps outline evidence-based interventions:

1. Eliminate the Trigger

Discontinue exposure to the allergen (e.g., medications, transfusions).

2. Airway Management

Ensure a clear airway; prepare for intubation if angioedema is present. Tracheostomy or cricothyroidotomy may be necessary in severe cases.

3. Oxygenation

Administer supplemental oxygen to maintain SpO2 >94–98%.

4. Circulation Support

For hypotension:

Adults: Rapid infusion of 1–2 liters of normal saline.

Children: Boluses of 20 mL/kg over 5–10 minutes, repeated as needed.

5. Patient Positioning

Supine position with elevated legs unless airway swelling or vomiting dictates otherwise. Pregnant patients should be positioned on their left side.

6. Adrenaline Administration

Intramuscular (IM) injection of 0.3–0.5 mg (1:1,000 dilution) in the anterolateral thigh, repeated every 5–15 minutes as necessary, up to three doses.

Dosage in children:

<6 years: 0.15 mg IM

6–12 years: 0.3 mg IM

> 12 years: 0.5 mg IM

Persistent hypotension: Administer intravenous (IV) adrenaline bolus (0.1–0.5 mg in 1:10,000 dilution) followed by infusion at 0.1 µg/kg/min.

7. Antihistamines

H1 blockers:

Chlorpheniramine 1–2 mL IV/IM

Promethazine 25 mg IV/IM

H2 blockers:

Ranitidine 50 mg IV, given every 8 hours.

8. Adjunctive Therapies

Hydrocortisone: 100–200 mg IV to prevent biphasic reactions.

Bronchodilators: Nebulized salbutamol (5 mg in 5 mL saline) for persistent bronchospasm.

Glucagon: 1–5 mg IV over 5 minutes, followed by infusion (5–15 µg/min) in β-blocker-dependent patients.

Observation and Discharge

Patients with mild symptoms should be observed for 4–6 hours before discharge. Stable patients can be discharged with the following prescriptions:

Levocetirizine: 5–10 mg once daily for 3–5 days

Ranitidine: 150 mg twice daily for 3–5 days

Prednisolone: 0.5 mg/kg once daily for 3 days

Key Considerations

Epinephrine remains the first-line treatment for anaphylaxis due to its ability to reverse airway obstruction and cardiovascular collapse. It should never be substituted with hydrocortisone in acute settings.

Steroids are administered to prevent delayed or prolonged reactions but are ineffective for immediate symptom relief.

By adhering to these guidelines, healthcare providers can effectively manage anaphylaxis and improve patient outcomes.

Chapter 4
Overview of Shock

Definition

Shock is a critical condition characterized by inadequate tissue perfusion and oxygen delivery, resulting in cellular and tissue hypoxia. This can stem from either diminished oxygen delivery to tissues or heightened oxygen consumption.

Classification of Shock

Shock can be classified into the following types based on the underlying mechanism:

1. Distributive Shock: Common examples include septic shock, neurogenic shock, anaphylactic shock, toxic shock syndrome, and Addisonian crisis.

2. Cardiogenic Shock: Caused by conditions such as myocardial infarction, arrhythmias, or structural damage like valve rupture or ventricular septal defect.

3. Hypovolemic Shock: Results from blood or fluid loss due to hemorrhage, diarrhea, vomiting, burns, or heatstroke.

4. Obstructive Shock: Caused by physical obstructions such as pulmonary embolism, tension pneumothorax, pulmonary hypertension, constrictive pericarditis, or restrictive cardiomyopathy.

Stages of Shock

1. Preshock (Compensated Shock): Early compensatory mechanisms like tachycardia and peripheral vasoconstriction attempt to maintain tissue perfusion. Prompt recognition and intervention at this stage can reverse the condition.

2. Shock (Decompensated Stage): Compensatory responses fail, leading to signs of organ dysfunction. Symptoms include hypotension, restlessness, tachycardia, metabolic acidosis, dyspnea, reduced urine output, cold clammy skin, and diaphoresis.

3. End Stage (Irreversible Shock): Persistent hypoperfusion results in multi-organ failure and irreversible damage. Patients often become comatose, progressing to death if untreated.

Vasopressors and Inotropes

Vasopressors and inotropes play a crucial role in managing shock by improving blood pressure and cardiac output.

Vasopressors: Agents like noradrenaline, adrenaline, and phenylephrine enhance vascular tone by inducing vasoconstriction.

Inotropes: Drugs such as dopamine and dobutamine improve myocardial contractility.

Key examples of these medications include:

Noradrenaline: Frequently used as the first-line agent in septic, cardiogenic, and hypovolemic shock, with side effects like hyperglycemia and bradyarrhythmias.

Adrenaline: Essential in anaphylactic shock and used as an adjunct in septic shock. Adverse effects include tachyarrhythmias, ischemia, and hyperglycemia.

Dopamine: Serves as a secondary agent in cardiogenic and septic shock but may cause arrhythmias.

Dobutamine: Often employed in cardiogenic shock and myocardial dysfunction, with potential risks of hypotension and tachyarrhythmias.

Management Principles

Shock management requires early identification and targeted interventions tailored to the underlying cause. General strategies include:

Hypovolemic Shock: Prioritize fluid resuscitation with intravenous (IV) fluids and blood products for hemorrhagic causes.

Septic Shock: Begin empiric antibiotic therapy promptly, ensure adequate fluid replacement, and use vasopressors such as noradrenaline to restore perfusion.

Cardiogenic Shock: Administer inotropic support, including adrenaline or dobutamine, to enhance cardiac output.

Obstructive Shock: Resolve physical obstructions through interventions like pericardiocentesis, thrombolysis, or needle thoracostomy.

Neurogenic Shock: Employ fluid resuscitation and vasopressors such as dopamine or noradrenaline to restore vascular tone.

Adrenal Crisis: Administer IV glucocorticoids alongside fluid resuscitation and supportive inotropic therapy as needed.

Key Considerations

In hypovolemic shock, restore intravascular volume with IV fluids before initiating vasopressors to avoid exacerbating tissue hypoperfusion. Certain subcutaneous drugs like heparin and insulin may show reduced efficacy due to vasoconstriction.

A structured approach with precise interventions tailored to the shock subtype ensures better patient outcomes. Recognizing and addressing the early stages of shock is critical in preventing progression to irreversible organ damage.

Chapter 5
Septic Shock

Introduction

Sepsis represents a severe medical condition resulting from a dysregulated immune response to infection, leading to systemic inflammation. It progresses from early-stage sepsis to the potentially fatal state of septic shock.

The systemic inflammatory response syndrome (SIRS) is a clinical reaction that can arise due to infectious or non-infectious causes. When associated with a suspected infection, it is classified as sepsis.

Systemic Inflammatory Response Syndrome (SIRS)
SIRS is traditionally identified through the following criteria:

Temperature >38.3°C or <36°C

Heart rate exceeding 90 beats per minute

Respiratory rate greater than 20 breaths per minute

White blood cell count >12,000/mm³ or <4,000/mm³

However, this definition has become outdated due to its limited sensitivity and specificity.

The 2016 Third International Consensus Definitions (Sepsis-3) redefined sepsis as life-threatening organ dysfunction caused by an imbalanced host response to infection. Organ dysfunction is indicated by an increase in the Sequential Organ Failure Assessment (SOFA) score by two or more points due to infection, correlating with a hospital mortality rate of approximately 10%.

Septic shock is a more critical condition characterized by severe circulatory, cellular, and metabolic abnormalities. It is identified by persistent hypotension requiring vasopressors to maintain a mean arterial pressure (MAP) above 65 mmHg and a serum lactate level above 2 mmol/L, even after adequate fluid resuscitation. Mortality in such cases exceeds 40%. The term "severe sepsis" is no longer used.

qSOFA and SOFA Scoring Systems
Predictive scoring systems such as the Quick Sequential Organ Failure Assessment (qSOFA) and SOFA help evaluate disease severity and outcomes, particularly mortality.

For patients suspected of sepsis, qSOFA is a simple bedside tool assessing three criteria:

Respiratory rate >22 breaths per minute

Altered mental state

Systolic blood pressure <100 mmHg

A score of two or more suggests a poor prognosis and warrants further investigation using the SOFA score. The SOFA score measures organ dysfunction to guide treatment and prioritize intensive care or specialized referrals. A higher SOFA score indicates worse patient outcomes.

National Early Warning Score 2 (NEWS2)
NEWS2 is another clinical scoring system designed to detect and respond to deterioration in acutely ill patients. It evaluates six parameters:

Respiratory rate

Oxygen saturation

Systolic blood pressure

Pulse rate

Consciousness level

Temperature

Patients with a NEWS2 score of five or more, combined with signs of infection, should be evaluated for sepsis.

Management of Severe Sepsis and Septic Shock

Septic shock requires aggressive management in the resuscitation phase, focusing on four critical interventions: fluid resuscitation, antibiotic therapy, source control, and temperature regulation.

Fluid Resuscitation

Administer crystalloids such as normal saline or Ringer's lactate at 10–20 mL/kg per bolus (up to 30 mL/kg) within the first hour, assessing response to treatment after each bolus.

A restrictive fluid approach may reduce mechanical ventilation duration and ICU stays, especially in patients with acute respiratory distress syndrome (ARDS).

For patients with persistent hypotension, vasopressors such as norepinephrine are first-line agents. Secondary vasopressors, including epinephrine or vasopressin, may be added to maintain MAP above 65 mmHg.

Antibiotic Therapy

Broad-spectrum antibiotics should be administered within the first hour of emergency department admission, following blood cultures from two distinct sites.

Preferred regimens include piperacillin-tazobactam for stable patients or meropenem for those in shock.

Control of Infection Source

Infection control involves identifying and removing the source of sepsis, such as abscesses, diabetic foot infections, or gastrointestinal perforations.

Temperature Management

Fever should be managed through external cooling methods and antipyretic medications to stabilize the patient.

Additional Measures

Hyperglycemia: Blood glucose levels should be maintained below 200 mg/dL.

Blood transfusion: Recommended when hemoglobin levels drop below 7 g/dL.

Lactate clearance: Monitoring lactate levels every six hours is essential to evaluate resuscitation efficacy.

Regular arterial blood gas analysis is crucial for assessing oxygen levels, acid-base balance, and potential complications like pulmonary edema or acute respiratory distress syndrome.

This structured approach ensures a comprehensive and evidence-based management strategy for septic shock, aiming to improve survival rates and clinical outcomes.

Chapter 6
Airway Management in the Emergency Department

Managing airways in the emergency department (ED) presents significant challenges due to the critical condition of patients and limited preparation time. Consequently, all airways should be assumed to be difficult, and a difficult airway management cart must always be readily available.

Airway Assessment in Emergency Settings

Emergency physicians can utilize specific mnemonics to anticipate potential airway difficulties. Two commonly used mnemonics are MOANS, for assessing difficulties with mask ventilation, and LEMON, for predicting challenges in laryngoscopy.

Assessing Difficult Mask Ventilation: MOANS

M – Mask seal: Issues such as facial injuries, beards, or blood can compromise the seal.

O – Obesity/obstruction: Obese patients or those with airway obstructions can be difficult to ventilate effectively with a mask.

A – Age (>55 years): Aging reduces airway compliance, complicating mask ventilation.

N – No teeth: Edentulous patients lack structural support, making mask sealing problematic.

S – Stiff lungs: Conditions like chronic obstructive pulmonary disease (COPD) or asthma result in stiff lungs, hindering mask ventilation.

Assessing a Difficult Airway: LEMON

1. L – Look externally: Identify any visible abnormalities, such as facial deformities, burns,

injuries, or thick facial hair, that may complicate intubation.

2. E – Evaluate the 3-3-2 rule:

Three fingerbreadths for mouth opening: Indicates adequate temporomandibular joint mobility.

Three fingerbreadths between mentum and hyoid bone: Demonstrates sufficient mandibular space to accommodate the tongue during laryngoscopy.

Two fingerbreadths between thyroid cartilage and hyoid bone: Absence may suggest a high or anterior larynx, which can be hard to visualize.

3. M – Mallampati score: Evaluates the anatomical structures visible when the patient opens their mouth while seated.

Grade 1: Easy airway.

Grade 4: Significantly challenging airway.

4. O – Obesity/obstruction: Look for anatomical obstructions, such as foreign bodies or stridor, indicating restricted airflow.

5. N – Neck mobility: Assess the patient's ability to flex and extend their neck. Limited mobility, common in conditions like diabetes, can make aligning airway structures for intubation difficult.

Additional Considerations

Dentures: Leave dentures in place during mask ventilation to enhance the seal. Remove them immediately before intubation to prevent dislodgement or aspiration.

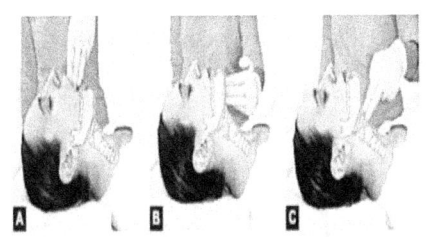

Figure 6-1A to C: Evaluating the 332 rule

Identification of a Compromised Airway

The identification of a compromised airway is critical in emergency settings to ensure timely intervention and prevent respiratory failure. Specific clinical signs and conditions should alert healthcare providers to potential airway obstruction or difficulty.

Clinical Signs of a Compromised Airway

The following signs indicate a compromised or obstructed airway:

Inspiratory stridor: A high-pitched sound indicating upper airway obstruction.

Gurgling: Suggestive of fluid, blood, or secretions obstructing the airway.

Snoring: Indicates partial airway obstruction, often due to soft tissue collapse.

Tracheal tug and subcostal retractions: Signs of increased effort to breathe, typically seen with airway obstruction.

Hoarseness or expiratory phonation: Suggests vocal cord involvement or upper airway narrowing.

Paradoxical chest wall movement: Chest and abdomen moving in opposite directions, a sign of severe airway compromise.

Rapid, shallow breathing: Indicates respiratory distress.

Central cyanosis: A late sign of hypoxemia, reflecting inadequate oxygenation.

Scenarios Associated with a Difficult Airway

Certain clinical conditions are known to predispose patients to a challenging airway. These include:

1. Maxillofacial trauma: Obstruction from bleeding, soft tissue swelling, or fractured bone segments.

2. Burns: Acute airway compromise due to glottic or tracheobronchial edema, restricted neck mobility, or reduced mouth opening from contractures.

3. Neoplasms: Tumors of the larynx or oral cavity causing airway narrowing or obstruction.

4. Arthritis: Conditions like temporomandibular joint arthritis or ankylosing spondylitis limit neck and jaw mobility, complicating airway management.

5. Infections: Severe infections causing airway inflammation or obstruction, such as:

Croup: Viral-induced upper airway obstruction in children.

Supraglottitis: Inflammation of the supraglottic structures.

Quinsy (Peritonsillar abscess): Swelling that can obstruct the oropharynx.

Retropharyngeal abscess: A deep neck infection that compresses the airway.

Ludwig's angina: Submandibular infection causing airway obstruction.

Angioedema: Rapid swelling of the airway due to allergic or idiopathic causes.

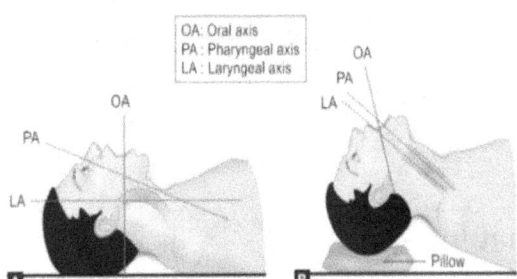

Figure 6-2A & B: Positioning of a patient during intubation

Preparation for Endotracheal Intubation

Effective preparation is critical for successful endotracheal (ET) intubation. Ensure the following steps are completed before proceeding:

Optimal Positioning

Position the neck in flexion and the head in extension to align the airway axes.

Use a pillow or folded sheet (approximately 10 cm in height) beneath the occiput in adults to elevate the head.

Essential Equipment

Prepare all necessary tools, including a bag-valve mask, suction catheter, ET tube, syringe, laryngoscope, laryngeal mask airway, bougie, and stylet.

Medication Preparation

Administer medications as per the established intubation protocol.

Team Communication

Ensure clear communication with the medical team to coordinate efforts effectively during the procedure.

Alignment of Airway Axes

To facilitate intubation, the path from the incisor teeth to the larynx should be as straight as possible. The alignment of the following axes is key:

1. The angle between the mouth and the larynx is 90 degrees.

2. The pharyngeal-to-tracheal angle is obtuse.

Raising the head approximately 10 cm using a folded sheet helps align the pharyngeal and laryngeal axes in most non-obese patients. Once aligned, extend the head using your right hand to optimize visualization of the airway.

Special Considerations

Cervical Spine Stability: For patients with suspected or confirmed cervical spine instability, manual in-line stabilization is essential to prevent further injury.

Obese Patients: Use a ramped position by placing pillows or sheets under the shoulders and upper torso to improve alignment and airway access.

Laryngeal Visualization – Cormack and Lehane Grading

The Cormack and Lehane grading system describes the view of the larynx during direct laryngoscopy:

Grade I: Full view of the vocal cords.

Grade II: Partial view of the cords or arytenoids.

Grade III: Only the epiglottis is visible.

Grade IV: Neither the epiglottis nor vocal cords are visible.

Accurate grading during intubation assists in assessing difficulty and ensuring appropriate adjustments to technique.

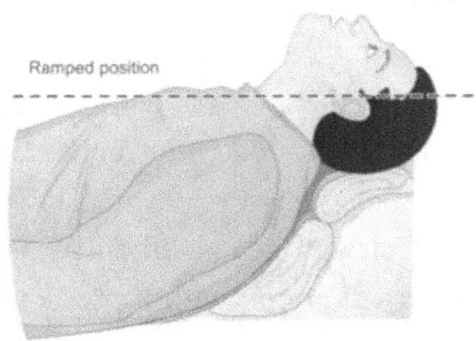

Figure 6-3: Ramped position.

Laryngeal Mask Airway (LMA)

The laryngeal mask airway (LMA) is a supraglottic device designed to sit within the hypopharynx, providing partial isolation of the trachea to facilitate positive pressure ventilation. It serves as an alternative to endotracheal intubation in both emergency department (ED) and prehospital settings under the following conditions:

1. Short Procedures: Suitable for brief interventions where neuromuscular blockade is not required.

2. Airway Rescue: Used as a rescue airway device in cases of failed endotracheal intubation.[1]

3. Difficult Airway Management: Enables blind intubation in situations with a predicted difficult airway, especially when advanced or alternative equipment is unavailable.

Size Selection

LMA devices are available in sizes ranging from 0 (for infants) to 5 (for adults weighing over 80 kg). The commonly recommended sizes for adults are:

Size 3 for adult females.

Size 4 for adult males.

Proper selection and placement of the LMA are critical to ensuring effective ventilation and patient safety during use.

References

Walls RM, Murphy MF. Manual of Emergency Airway Management, 3rd Edition. Philadelphia: Lippincott, Williams, and Wilkins; 2009, pp. 9-10.

Chapter 7
Respiratory Support

Introduction

Oxygen therapy is a cornerstone of respiratory support and can be delivered effectively through various oronasal devices such as nasal cannulas, catheters, or masks. Appropriate selection and use of these devices are critical in managing patients with compromised respiratory function.

Oxygen Delivery Methods

Face Masks: Equipped with oxygen flow meters or Venturi mechanisms, these masks ensure controlled oxygen delivery.

FiO_2 Calculation: The inspired oxygen fraction (FiO_2) is determined using the formula: FiO_2 (%) = 20 + (4 × O_2 flow rate in L/min).

SpO_2 and PaO_2 Correlation: A PaO_2 of 60 mmHg corresponds to an SpO_2 of approximately 90%. However, in conditions such as metabolic acidosis, a higher PaO_2 target is necessary.

Flow Rate Adjustments by Device:

Nasal Cannula: Oxygen flow rate up to 4 L/min.

Simple Face Mask: Oxygen flow rate of 6–10 L/min.

Venturi Mask: Oxygen flow rate of 2–15 L/min.

Non-Rebreather Mask with Reservoir Bag: Oxygen flow rate of 10–15 L/min.

Potential Risks of Oxygen Therapy

1. Physical Risks: High oxygen concentrations increase the risk of fire hazards and tank explosions. Dry, non humidified oxygen can lead to nasal and oral mucosal dryness and crusting.

2. Functional Risks: In patients with conditions like chronic obstructive pulmonary disease (COPD), reliance on hypoxic drive for breathing can result in ventilatory depression if excessive oxygen is administered.

3. Cytotoxic Effects: High oxygen concentrations can release reactive oxygen species (ROS), potentially causing lung tissue damage at a structural level.

Types of Respiratory Failure

1. Type 1 Respiratory Failure: Defined by a PaO_2 < 8 kPa (60 mmHg), typically with normal or reduced $PaCO_2$ levels. It indicates oxygenation failure.

2. Type 2 Respiratory Failure: Characterized by hypercapnia (elevated $PaCO_2$), with or without hypoxia, indicating ventilatory failure.

Ventilatory Support Modalities

Noninvasive Ventilation (NIV)

Noninvasive ventilation provides positive pressure support via masks or nasal prongs, avoiding the need for invasive devices such as endotracheal tubes. It is beneficial for both oxygenation and ventilation support.

Modes of NIV

1. Noninvasive Positive Pressure Ventilation (NIPPV): Delivered via standard ventilators or specialized machines such as CPAP or BiPAP.

2. Continuous Positive Airway Pressure (CPAP): Often used in oxygenation failure, such as pulmonary edema.

3. Bilevel Positive Airway Pressure (BiPAP): Used for ventilation failure, such as in hypercapnic respiratory conditions.

Indications for NIV

Acute exacerbation of COPD with respiratory acidosis.

Cardiogenic pulmonary edema resistant to medical therapy.

Hypercapnic respiratory failure due to chest wall deformities or neuromuscular conditions.

Post-extubation weaning or management of decompensated obstructive sleep apnea.

Contraindications for NIV

Comatose patients (Glasgow Coma Scale <8).

Airway obstruction or extensive facial trauma.

Patients with unstable hemodynamics requiring multiple inotropes.

Conditions like significant secretions, recent upper gastrointestinal surgery, vomiting, or respiratory arrest.

BiPAP Initial Settings

IPAP (Inspiratory Positive Airway Pressure): Start at 15 cm H_2O, increase up to 20 cm H_2O if tolerated.

EPAP (Expiratory Positive Airway Pressure): Set at 5 cm H_2O. Adjust gradually for optimal ventilation and oxygenation.

Key Notes:

Monitor FiO_2 adjustments carefully when increasing pressures on BiPAP.

Ensure a well-fitted interface to minimize leaks and maintain patient comfort.

Invasive Ventilation

Reserved for patients with severe respiratory compromise who fail to respond to noninvasive methods.

Indications for Intubation

Cardiac arrest or apnea.

GCS <8 in trauma.

Persistent hypoxemia (SpO_2 <90%) despite NIV.

Impending respiratory arrest or elective management in specific conditions (e.g., tetanus).

Ventilator Initial Settings

Mode: SIMV (Synchronized Intermittent Mandatory Ventilation), volume-controlled with pressure support.

FiO_2: 100% initially, titrate to SpO_2 targets.

PEEP: 5 cm H_2O; increase gradually to maintain oxygenation.

Tidal Volume: 6–8 mL/kg body weight.

Rate: 10–15 breaths/min.

Pressure Support: 12 cm H_2O.

Monitoring Requirements:

Regular ABG evaluations to assess gas exchange and ventilator settings.

Ensure peak and plateau pressures remain within safe limits (peak <35 cm H_2O, plateau <30 cm H_2O).

Monitor for complications such as pneumothorax, tube obstruction, or ventilator-associated lung injuries.

Key Management Points:

Adequate sedation using agents like midazolam is essential to ensure patient comfort and synchrony with the ventilator.

Avoid neuromuscular blocking agents unless absolutely necessary, ensuring proper sedation beforehand.

Optimize hydration to prevent hypotension, especially in conditions like Guillain–Barré syndrome.

Special Considerations

Oxygenation improvement can be achieved by adjusting FiO_2, PEEP, and recruitment maneuvers.

Ventilation adjustments (for CO_2 regulation) involve modifying tidal volume and respiratory rate.

Address the underlying pathology (e.g., bronchodilators in asthma) for improved outcomes.

This structured approach ensures the effective application of respiratory support tailored to patient needs, emphasizing safety, precision, and evidence-based practices.

Section 3
Fluid and Electrolyte Management

Chapter 8
Fluid Therapy
Overview and Applications

Introduction

Water accounts for approximately 60% of the human body weight, with the remaining 40% consisting of lean body mass. The body's water is distributed across two primary compartments: intracellular and extracellular. The extracellular compartment is further divided into the interstitial fluid and plasma (intravascular space). These compartments maintain a dynamic balance, with fluid and electrolyte exchanges occurring across membranes, ensuring fluid homeostasis (Fig. 1).

Choice of Intravenous Fluids

In the emergency department, various crystalloids and colloids are utilized for fluid resuscitation. These fluids are distributed across both intracellular and extracellular compartments, as outlined in Table 1. A breakdown of commonly used crystalloids is provided in Table 2. The appropriate selection of intravenous fluids depends on the clinical condition and the desired effect on the patient's fluid compartments.

1. Normal Saline (0.9% NS)

Normal saline is an isotonic crystalloid commonly used in trauma cases and for dehydrated patients. It primarily expands the extracellular fluid volume without altering the intracellular volume. However, excessive use may lead to hyperchloremic acidosis, particularly in large volumes.

2. Ringer Lactate (RL)

Ringer lactate is another isotonic crystalloid frequently used in the management of acute gastroenteritis (AGE). It expands extracellular volume, with minimal effect on the intravascular volume. Caution should be exercised in patients with diabetic ketoacidosis (DKA) due to the potential for elevated serum lactate levels.

3. Dextrose Normal Saline (DNS)
This solution is a mixed crystalloid used when resuscitation is needed alongside calorie replacement, particularly in postoperative patients with low blood sugar. It helps provide both fluid and energy, but it may not be suitable in all clinical situations due to its potential effects on electrolyte balance.

4. 5% Dextrose
Although not commonly used for initial resuscitation, 5% dextrose is appropriate for managing free water deficits in patients with hypernatremia. It is primarily used for infusions requiring a solvent, such as noradrenaline. However, it can lead to complications like hyponatremia, cerebral edema, pulmonary

edema, hyperglycemia, and hypokalemia if not carefully monitored.

5. Hypotonic Saline Solutions (1/2 NS, 1/4 NS)

These solutions are utilized for correcting free water deficits in hypernatremic patients. While effective, they carry risks such as hyponatremia and cerebral or pulmonary edema, particularly in patients with compromised renal or cardiac function.

6. Hypertonic Saline (3% NaCl)

3% NaCl is a hypertonic crystalloid that expands extracellular volume and reduces intracellular volume. It is used in cases of severe hyponatremia and cerebral edema. Although effective in these critical conditions, it can lead to osmotic demyelination syndrome if administered too rapidly or in excessive amounts.

Fluid Distribution and Effects

Table 1 outlines the net effect of infusing 500 mL of various fluids on the intracellular and extracellular compartments. For example, normal saline mainly impacts extracellular fluid, with minimal effect on intracellular volume. Conversely, dextrose solutions and colloids have different distribution patterns, which should be considered when selecting fluids for specific clinical scenarios.

Crystalloid Composition

Table 2 compares the composition of commonly used crystalloid solutions. Key parameters include sodium (Na), chloride (Cl), bicarbonate (HCO_3), osmolarity (mOsm), and pH. This composition plays a critical role in determining the fluid's effect on the body's electrolytes and its ability to maintain proper fluid balance.

By understanding the physiological roles and effects of these fluids, healthcare providers can make informed decisions on fluid therapy, ensuring that the patient receives the most appropriate resuscitation based on their clinical condition.

Chapter 9
Sodium

Introduction

This chapter explores sodium, a vital electrolyte, whose normal serum concentration ranges from 135–145 mEq/L.

Hyponatremia

Hyponatremia is characterized by a serum sodium level below 135 mmol/L. Its symptoms include headache, nausea, vomiting, fatigue, confusion, gait disturbances, seizures, and, in severe cases, coma or respiratory arrest. Table 1 outlines its causes and management.

Pseudohyponatremia: Conditions like hyperglycemia, hyperproteinemia, and hypertriglyceridemia can artificially lower sodium levels. Correction involves addressing glucose or BUN levels using specified formulas.

Management Guidelines:

Sodium correction must proceed cautiously, avoiding an increase of more than 10–12 mmol/L in 24 hours to prevent complications such as central pontine myelinolysis.

Severe hyponatremia (Na <120 mEq/L) or symptomatic cases (e.g., seizures) may require 3% NaCl infusion but only under euvolemic or dilutional states.

Diagnostic tools include urine and serum osmolality and spot urine sodium to differentiate true hyponatremia from pseudohyponatremia.

Hypernatremia

Hypernatremia occurs when serum sodium exceeds 145 mEq/L, often due to water deficits or excessive sodium intake. Causes are categorized as excess sodium (e.g., hypertonic saline administration) or relative water deficiency (e.g., diabetes insipidus).

Management:

Sodium reduction should not exceed 10–12 mEq/L daily to prevent neurologic complications.

Fluids like 5% dextrose, ½ NS, or free water are administered based on glucose levels and patient tolerance.

The Adrogue–Madias formula is used to calculate water deficits for appropriate correction.

Chapter 10
Potassium

Introduction

Potassium, a predominantly intracellular ion, has normal serum levels between 3.5–5 mEq/L. Its balance is influenced by acidosis (causing hyperkalemia) and alkalosis (leading to hypokalemia).

Hypokalemia

Low potassium levels, often resulting from gastrointestinal losses, diuretic use, or redistribution, manifest as muscle weakness, fatigue, or constipation. Severe cases can lead to significant cardiac arrhythmias, reflected as T wave inversion and U waves on ECG.

Management:

Potassium replacement varies depending on the deficit, with larger doses required at lower serum levels.

Magnesium supplementation is crucial in cases of severe hypokalemia (<3 mEq/L), especially for patients on diuretics or digoxin.

Long-term management includes syrup potassium chloride and addressing underlying causes like diuretic therapy.

Hyperkalemia

Hyperkalemia, or elevated potassium levels (>5 mEq/L), arises from increased intake, reduced excretion (e.g., renal failure), or intracellular potassium shifts due to acidosis or tissue damage.

Treatment Strategies

1. Cardioprotection: Calcium gluconate stabilizes myocardial membranes.

2. Intracellular Shift: Insulin with dextrose and nebulized salbutamol drive potassium back into cells.

3. Excretion: Furosemide, potassium-binding resins, or hemodialysis remove potassium from the body.

Monitoring potassium levels post-correction is critical to prevent recurrence.

Chapter 11
Calcium

Introduction

Calcium exists in three forms in circulation:

1. Protein-bound (40–50%).

2. Ionized (40–45%), the physiologically active fraction.

3. Non-ionized chelated forms (10–15%).

Hypocalcemia

This condition, marked by ionized calcium levels below the normal range, presents with symptoms such as muscle cramps, tetany, paresthesia, and cardiac arrhythmias. Chvostek's and Trousseau's signs are hallmark findings.

Management:

Acute hypocalcemia is managed with intravenous calcium gluconate.

Chronic conditions may require vitamin D supplementation and dietary calcium intake.

Hypercalcemia

Hypercalcemia, with serum calcium >10.5 mg/dL, often results from malignancies or primary hyperparathyroidism. Symptoms include nausea, fatigue, polyuria, and confusion.

Management:

Immediate hydration with saline promotes calcium excretion.

Medications such as bisphosphonates, calcitonin, or corticosteroids lower calcium levels in resistant cases.

Chapter 12
Magnesium

Introduction

Magnesium is an essential mineral, with normal serum levels ranging from 1.7–2.2 mg/dL. It is vital for neuromuscular function and enzyme activity.

Hypomagnesemia

Deficiency (<1.7 mg/dL) can stem from malabsorption, chronic alcoholism, or renal losses. Clinical features include muscle tremors, seizures, and cardiac arrhythmias such as torsades de pointes.

Treatment:

Intravenous magnesium sulfate is administered for acute deficits.

Oral magnesium supplements are used for mild or chronic deficiencies.

Hypermagnesemia

Excess magnesium (>2.2 mg/dL), often linked to renal failure or excessive intake, manifests as hypotension, bradycardia, or respiratory depression.

Management:

Intravenous calcium gluconate counteracts the cardiac effects.

Dialysis is employed in severe cases to reduce magnesium levels.

Chapter 13
Acid-Base Abnormalities

Introduction

The assessment of acid-base disorders begins with a thorough history and physical examination of the patient. The following are normal reference ranges for key parameters:

pH: 7.35–7.45

PaCO2: 35–45 mm Hg

HCO3: 22–26 mmol/L

PaO2: >60 mm Hg (typically 80–100 mm Hg)

A correlation exists between SpO2 and PaO2, but below 90% SpO2, PaO2 declines more sharply than SpO2 levels.

Respiratory acidosis/alkalosis is compensated by the kidneys, which take longer to respond.

Metabolic acidosis/alkalosis is compensated by the lungs, with a faster response time.

It is essential to note that compensatory mechanisms never overcorrect. For instance, a metabolic acidosis prompts the lungs to eliminate CO_2, but the compensation will not result in respiratory alkalosis.

Compensation Rules for Metabolic Disorders

In cases of metabolic acidosis or alkalosis, compensation involves a corresponding drop or rise in $PaCO_2$. The adjusted $PaCO_2$ value is expected to fall within ±5 mm Hg of the digits following the decimal point of the pH value, provided the pH remains between 7.1 and 7.6.

Compensation Rules for Respiratory Disorders

For respiratory disorders, compensation occurs via renal mechanisms, which act more slowly. Acute events display less compensation compared to chronic conditions. If the pH is within the normal range but PaCO2 and HCO3 levels are abnormal, a mixed acid-base disorder should be suspected.

Interpreting Arterial Blood Gas (ABG) Results

1. Obtain a detailed history to identify the primary metabolic or respiratory issue.

2. Evaluate PaO2 and calculate the PaO2/FiO2 ratio to optimize oxygen levels.

3. Assess the pH:

A pH <7.3 indicates acidosis.

A pH >7.5 indicates alkalosis.

If the pH is normal but CO2 or HCO3 is abnormal, consider a mixed disorder.

4. Examine base excess (BE):

BE < –2 indicates metabolic acidosis.

BE > +2 indicates metabolic alkalosis.

5. Apply compensation rules to evaluate if the response aligns with the expected compensatory mechanism.

6. Calculate the anion gap for metabolic acidosis:

Formula: (Na + K) – (HCO3 + Cl)

Normal range: 14 ± 4.

7. Review electrolytes and glucose for abnormalities and correct as needed.

8. Investigate lactate and methemoglobin levels for additional diagnostic clues and address the underlying cause.

Comparison of ABG and Venous Blood Gas (VBG) Analysis

pH: Venous pH closely mirrors arterial pH in most metabolic conditions except during cardiac arrest, where differences increase as cardiac output decreases.

Lactate: Arterial and venous lactate levels are comparable, especially when elevated (>2 mmol/L). A normal venous lactate level reliably predicts normal arterial levels.

HCO3: Similar values are observed in ABG and VBG.

PaCO2: Venous PaCO2 is typically higher than arterial PaCO2, making VBG insufficient for determining hypercarbia.

PaO2: Venous PaO2 does not correlate with arterial PaO2 and is therefore unreliable for assessing oxygen delivery.

Clinical Utility of ABG and VBG

In most cases, a detailed history and physical examination provide more insight than ABG or VBG results. Dependency on ABG should be minimized except in specific clinical scenarios.

Indications for VBG

Diabetic ketoacidosis (DKA) to determine pH and lactate levels.

Acute severe pancreatitis with shock.

Renal failure to assess pH and dialysis requirements.

Detecting electrolyte abnormalities (e.g., potassium or magnesium) in arrhythmias or impending cardiac arrest.

Indications for ABG

Although VBG is simpler and provides most essential information, ABG is required in specific situations:

Chronic obstructive pulmonary disease (COPD) exacerbation with suspected type 2 respiratory failure to assess $PaCO_2$ and determine the need for ventilation.

Type 1 respiratory failure in patients on noninvasive ventilation (NIV) or mechanical ventilation to adjust oxygen flow rates.

High-flow oxygen therapy patients to calculate PaO_2/FiO_2 ratios and evaluate the need for invasive ventilation.

Summary

ABG should only be performed in critical situations requiring detailed arterial parameters, such as type 2 respiratory failure or high-flow oxygen therapy. For most other conditions, VBG provides sufficient diagnostic information and simplifies the process. Accurate interpretation combined with a strong clinical foundation ensures optimal management of acid-base disorders.

Section 4
Infectious Diseases

Chapter 14
Antibiotic Protocol for Common Conditions

Introduction

Infections and febrile illnesses are commonly encountered in the emergency department (ED). Proper antibiotic therapy is essential for treating bacterial infections, preventing complications, and improving patient outcomes. This chapter outlines the antibiotic protocol for a range of common infections, including gastroenteritis, cellulitis, and more severe conditions like septic arthritis and meningitis.

Acute Gastroenteritis

Most cases of acute gastroenteritis are caused by viruses and do not require antibiotics. However, bacterial infections like Vibrio cholerae and Shigella species may necessitate antibiotic treatment. For cholera, doxycycline is recommended, while ciprofloxacin is used for shigellosis.

Bacillary Dysentery
For Shigella infections, antibiotics are reserved for severe cases or immunocompromised patients. Ciprofloxacin is typically the first choice, while azithromycin is an alternative.

Giardiasis
Giardia lamblia causes giardiasis, which can be treated effectively with tinidazole or metronidazole.

Typhoid Fever
The mainstay of treatment for Salmonella or Salmonella infections is azithromycin, with ceftriaxone as an alternative for severe cases.

Cholangitis and Acute Cholecystitis
These conditions are usually caused by Enterobacteriaceae and anaerobic bacteria. Piperacillin-tazobactam is recommended for

their treatment, with cefoperazone-sulbactam as an alternative.

Cellulitis

Staphylococcus aureus and Streptococcus pyogenes are common culprits in cellulitis. Clindamycin and cefuroxime are effective treatment options, with oral antibiotics like cephalexin or cloxacillin for mild cases.

Necrotizing Fasciitis

Necrotizing fasciitis requires immediate, aggressive treatment. First-line antibiotics include meropenem combined with vancomycin, with piperacillin-tazobactam and clindamycin as alternatives.

Septic Arthritis

For septic arthritis, Staphylococcus aureus is the most common pathogen. First-line treatment includes cloxacillin or cefazolin. In cases of methicillin-resistant Staphylococcus aureus (MRSA), vancomycin is used.

Acute Meningitis

Empiric treatment for bacterial meningitis includes ceftriaxone, vancomycin, and dexamethasone. Ampicillin should be added if Listeria monocytogenes is suspected.

Dengue Fever

Dengue is primarily a viral infection, and antibiotics are not effective. Management focuses on symptomatic relief, fluid management, and monitoring for signs of severe dengue.

Chapter 15
Dengue

Introduction

Dengue is a viral disease transmitted by Aedes mosquitoes. It is characterized by a sudden onset of fever, severe headache, retro-orbital pain, and generalized muscle and joint pain. Severe forms of dengue can lead to hemorrhagic manifestations and shock. This chapter discusses the clinical presentation, diagnostic approaches, and management strategies for dengue.

Clinical Presentation and Case Definitions

Dengue Fever: Characterized by fever, myalgia, rash, and retro-orbital pain.

Dengue Hemorrhagic Fever (DHF): Defined by fever, hemorrhagic manifestations, and a drop in platelet count, potentially progressing to plasma leakage.

Dengue Shock Syndrome (DSS): A critical complication marked by hypotension, requiring immediate resuscitation.

Management Strategies

Supportive Care: Oral or intravenous fluids are critical in preventing dehydration.

Monitoring: Close monitoring of hematocrit and platelet levels is essential to identify severe cases.

Treatment: No specific antiviral treatment is available. The main focus is on symptomatic management, with platelet transfusions indicated for severe thrombocytopenia.

Chapter 16
Malaria

Introduction

Malaria is a parasitic infection transmitted by Anopheles mosquitoes, primarily caused by Plasmodium falciparum, Plasmodium , Plasmodium ovale, and Plasmodium . This chapter outlines the clinical presentation, diagnosis, and treatment of malaria.

Clinical Presentation

Malaria presents with cyclic fever, chills, sweating, and flu-like symptoms, often accompanied by anemia, jaundice, and splenomegaly. Severe malaria can lead to organ failure, coma, and death.

Diagnosis

Diagnosis is made via blood smear or rapid diagnostic tests (RDTs) that detect Plasmodium antigens. Polymerase chain reaction (PCR) can be used for more accurate species identification.

Treatment

First-line Treatment: Artemisinin-based combination therapy (ACT) is the standard for uncomplicated malaria caused by Plasmodium falciparum. Chloroquine or primaquine is used for infections with Plasmodium .

Severe Malaria: For severe cases, intravenous artesunate is recommended, followed by oral ACT once the patient stabilizes.

Chapter 17
Tuberculosis

Introduction

Tuberculosis (TB) is a chronic infectious disease caused by Mycobacterium tuberculosis. It primarily affects the lungs but can involve any organ system. This chapter provides an overview of the clinical features, diagnosis, and treatment of TB.

Clinical Presentation

Symptoms of TB include chronic cough, hemoptysis, weight loss, night sweats, and fever. Extrapulmonary TB can affect the lymph nodes, bones, and other organs.

Diagnosis

The diagnosis of TB is based on clinical features, chest X-rays, sputum smear microscopy, and culture. Nucleic acid amplification tests (NAAT) like the GeneXpert MTB/RIF are also used for rapid diagnosis.

Treatment

First-line Drugs: The standard treatment regimen includes rifampin, isoniazid, pyrazinamide, and ethambutol for a duration of 6 months.

Drug-Resistant TB: Multidrug-resistant TB (MDR-TB) requires second-line agents like fluoroquinolones and injectable drugs such as amikacin.

Chapter 18
Sepsis

Introduction

Sepsis is a life-threatening condition caused by an infection that leads to systemic inflammatory response syndrome (SIRS). This chapter discusses the pathophysiology, clinical features, diagnostic criteria, and management of sepsis.

Pathophysiology

Sepsis occurs when the body's response to an infection leads to widespread inflammation, resulting in tissue damage, organ dysfunction, and sometimes organ failure. The condition is characterized by altered blood flow, cellular dysfunction, and metabolic changes.

Clinical Presentation

Symptoms of sepsis include fever, chills, tachycardia, hypotension, and altered mental status. Patients may develop organ dysfunction, including acute kidney injury, respiratory failure, and coagulopathy.

Diagnosis

The diagnosis of sepsis is based on the presence of infection and signs of systemic inflammation, with laboratory tests showing elevated white blood cell count, lactate levels, and procalcitonin.

Management

Early Goal-Directed Therapy: This includes intravenous fluids, vasopressors, and antibiotics. Early administration of broad-spectrum antibiotics is critical.

Antibiotic Therapy: Empiric therapy should cover common pathogens, including Staphylococcus aureus, Escherichia coli, and

Streptococcus pneumoniae. Specific antibiotics should be adjusted based on culture results.

Supportive Care: Mechanical ventilation, renal replacement therapy, and other organ support measures may be necessary for critically ill patients.

Chapter 19
Influenza and H1N1

Introduction

Seasonal influenza, an acute respiratory infection caused by influenza A or B viruses, is highly contagious and spreads primarily via respiratory droplets. Influenza viruses are further classified based on their surface proteins: hemagglutinin (H) and neuraminidase (N).

The H1N1 strain of influenza A became prominent during the 2008 pandemic. While most cases are mild and self-limiting, certain individuals, especially those in high-risk groups, can develop severe complications. The incubation period of influenza is typically 1–4 days, and the infectious period lasts 3–5 days after symptoms begin.

Clinical Features

Symptoms commonly include fever, nasal congestion (coryza), sore throat, cough, breathlessness, muscle aches (myalgia), and throat redness. Severe cases may involve rapid breathing (tachypnea), widespread lung crackles (crepitations), low blood pressure (hypotension), low oxygen levels (hypoxemia), or respiratory failure.

Investigations

Diagnosis involves a combination of laboratory and radiological evaluations:

1. Blood tests, including complete blood count and renal/liver function panels, may show leukopenia, mild liver enzyme elevation, or increased urea nitrogen.

2. Chest X-rays may reveal lung consolidation or diffuse infiltrates in severe cases.

3. PCR testing of nasal or throat swabs is the gold standard for confirmation, though treatment initiation should not be delayed awaiting results.

High-Risk Groups

Severe disease and complications are more likely in:

Pregnant individuals.

Children under 2 years and adults over 65 years.

Patients with chronic conditions like heart disease or diabetes.

Immunocompromised individuals or those with HIV infection.

Individuals with obesity.

Management

Low-risk individuals typically require symptomatic treatment, including antipyretics, antihistamines, and cough suppressants. High-risk individuals or those with severe symptoms should receive antiviral therapy with oseltamivir within 48 hours of symptom onset. Severe respiratory failure may require oxygen therapy, mechanical ventilation, and antibiotics for secondary bacterial infections.

Post-Exposure Prophylaxis

Close contacts of confirmed cases, especially those at high risk, should receive oseltamivir prophylaxis within 48 hours of exposure to reduce the likelihood of infection.

Vaccination

Annual influenza vaccination is recommended for high-risk populations and healthcare workers. Administering the vaccine in the pre-peak season, such as October–November in the Northern Hemisphere, optimizes immunity.

Chapter 20
COVID-19

Introduction

Coronavirus Disease 2019 (COVID-19) is a respiratory illness caused by the SARS-CoV-2 virus, first identified in late 2019 in Wuhan, China. The disease spreads through respiratory droplets, direct contact, and fomites. The incubation period ranges from 2 to 14 days, with the infectious period typically lasting up to 10 days, though it may extend in severe cases.

Clinical Presentation

Symptoms of COVID-19 range widely, from asymptomatic infection to severe respiratory failure. Early symptoms include fever, cough, sore throat, muscle pain, fatigue, diarrhea, and a loss of taste or smell. Severe cases can progress to acute respiratory distress syndrome (ARDS), thromboembolic complications, and multi-organ failure, particularly in older adults or those with comorbidities.

Diagnostic Evaluation

RT-PCR testing of nasopharyngeal swabs remains the gold standard for COVID-19 diagnosis. Imaging studies such as chest X-rays and CT scans often reveal bilateral air-space opacities, ground-glass opacities, and peripheral or basal consolidations.

Management by Severity

Mild cases, characterized by stable oxygen levels and minimal symptoms, require home isolation, hydration, and symptomatic treatment. Moderate cases may need hospitalization for monitoring and supplemental oxygen if required. Severe or critical cases demand aggressive interventions, including corticosteroids, antiviral agents like remdesivir, oxygen therapy, prone positioning, and mechanical ventilation for respiratory failure. Broad-spectrum antibiotics may be necessary to treat secondary bacterial infections.

Prevention and Control

Preventive measures include frequent handwashing, the use of face masks, maintaining physical distance, and vaccination. Vaccines targeting SARS-CoV-2 have significantly reduced severe illness and mortality rates, making them essential for pandemic control.

Chapter 21
Vaccination Strategies for Emerging Respiratory Viruses

Introduction

Vaccination serves as a cornerstone in preventing and controlling respiratory viral infections. It reduces transmission, prevents complications, and alleviates the burden on healthcare systems during outbreaks.

Influenza Vaccination

Influenza vaccines, reformulated annually to match circulating strains, are recommended for high-risk groups such as pregnant women, young children, older adults, and individuals with chronic illnesses. Healthcare workers should also be vaccinated to protect vulnerable patients.

COVID-19 Vaccination

COVID-19 vaccines have been developed using diverse technologies, including mRNA, viral vector, and inactivated virus platforms. Vaccination programs prioritize high-risk populations and healthcare providers, with booster doses administered to sustain immunity, especially in light of emerging variants. Monitoring adverse events and ensuring equitable vaccine distribution are critical for public health success.

Challenges in Vaccination Efforts

Global challenges include vaccine hesitancy, logistical barriers in low-resource settings, and the rapid mutation of viruses, necessitating updated vaccines. Public education and international collaboration are essential to address these issues effectively.

Future Directions

Research into universal vaccines targeting conserved viral components is ongoing, offering hope for broader and longer-lasting immunity. Additionally, advancements in vaccine technology, such as nanoparticle-based platforms, hold promise for combating future pandemics.

Chapter 22
Food Poisoning and Acute Gastroenteritis

Introduction

Food poisoning arises from consuming food or water contaminated by bacteria, their toxins, viruses, parasites, or chemicals. Diarrheal conditions resulting from food poisoning are broadly classified into two categories: non-inflammatory and inflammatory diarrhea, based on the mechanism of action and involvement of the intestinal mucosa.

Non-inflammatory Diarrhea:
Caused by enterotoxin-producing organisms like Vibrio cholerae, enterotoxigenic Escherichia coli (ETEC), Clostridium perfringens, Bacillus cereus, and Staphylococcus aureus. Viruses such as rotavirus, Norwalk virus, and adenovirus, along with parasites like Giardia lamblia and Cryptosporidium, can also cause

non-inflammatory diarrhea by disrupting intestinal absorption without inducing mucosal inflammation.

Clinical Features: Watery diarrhea, absence of fever or blood in stools.

Inflammatory Diarrhea:
Induced by cytotoxin-producing organisms like Clostridium difficile and invasive pathogens such as Salmonella, Shigella, Campylobacter, and Entamoeba . These agents lead to mucosal inflammation or direct tissue invasion.

Clinical Features: Fever, bloody diarrhea, abdominal pain, and systemic symptoms.

Management

1. Hydration Therapy:

Oral Rehydration: For mild to moderate dehydration, use oral rehydration solutions (ORS), with 200 mL given after each loose stool. Home-based hydration alternatives include diluted fruit juices, soups, or sports drinks.

Intravenous Hydration: Severe dehydration or shock necessitates IV fluids. Administer Ringer's lactate via an 18-G cannula or, in pediatric patients, a 20 mL/kg bolus of normal saline (NS) or Ringer's lactate, repeating as necessary.

2. Symptomatic Management:

For vomiting: Administer ondansetron 8 mg IV.

If gastric discomfort occurs: Consider IV pantoprazole or omeprazole.

Monitor urine output for early signs of acute kidney injury and address electrolyte imbalances promptly.

3. Antibiotic Use:

Antibiotics are generally not required in most cases of acute gastroenteritis, but specific scenarios demand targeted therapy:

Cholera: Treat with doxycycline (300 mg once, then 100 mg twice daily for 3 days).

Bacillary Dysentery: Treat with azithromycin (1 g single dose) or ciprofloxacin (500 mg twice daily for 3 days).

Amoebiasis: Initiate metronidazole therapy following stool sample analysis.

4. Precautions:

Avoid antimotility agents like loperamide, particularly in suspected invasive or infectious diarrhea.

Etiology Based on Incubation Period

Very Short Incubation Period (1–6 Hours):

Pathogens: Bacillus cereus, Staphylococcus aureus.

Source: Improperly stored rice, meat, eggs, or salads.

Symptoms: Severe nausea and vomiting, with minimal diarrhea.

Management: Supportive care; antibiotics are not indicated.

Short Incubation Period (10–48 Hours):

Pathogens: Clostridium perfringens, Rotavirus, Norovirus.

Symptoms: Watery diarrhea and abdominal cramps.

Management: Supportive care only.

Long Incubation Period (1–5 Days):

Pathogens: Vibrio cholerae, Salmonella, Shigella, Campylobacter.

Symptoms: Diarrhea (often bloody in invasive cases), fever.

Management: Antibiotics required for cholera, bacillary dysentery, or severe infections.

Chapter 23
Urinary Tract Infections (UTI)

Introduction

Urinary tract infections (UTIs) encompass a spectrum of conditions caused by bacterial colonization in the urinary system, presenting with distinct symptoms based on the site of infection.

Lower UTI (Cystitis):

Symptoms: Dysuria, frequency, urgency, and suprapubic discomfort.

Absence of fever distinguishes cystitis from upper UTI.

Upper UTI (Pyelonephritis):

Symptoms: Fever, chills, flank pain, nausea, vomiting, and costovertebral angle tenderness.

Management

1. Uncomplicated UTI:

Cystitis:

Preferred antibiotics: Nitrofurantoin 100 mg four times daily for 5–7 days or ciprofloxacin 500 mg twice daily for 3 days.

Alternatives: Trimethoprim-sulfamethoxazole (TMP-SMX).

Pyelonephritis:

Outpatient: Oral fluoroquinolones (e.g., ciprofloxacin).

Severe Cases: Hospitalization and IV antibiotics (e.g., ceftriaxone, piperacillin-tazobactam).

2. Complicated UTI:

Requires hospitalization for IV carbapenems (e.g., meropenem 1 g every 8 hours).

3. Asymptomatic Bacteriuria:

Treatment indicated only in pregnant women or patients undergoing urologic procedures likely to cause mucosal bleeding.

Diagnostic Investigations

Urinalysis:

Significant findings: >5 WBCs in males or >10 in females.

Positive leukocyte esterase or nitrite test confirms infection.

Imaging:

Ultrasonography is indicated for unresponsive cases, structural abnormalities, or suspected renal stones.

Chapter 24
Acute Central Nervous System (CNS) Infections

Introduction

Acute CNS infections include meningitis, encephalitis, and brain abscesses, each involving distinct pathophysiology and clinical presentations.

Meningitis: Inflammation of the meninges, primarily caused by Streptococcus pneumoniae or Neisseria .

Symptoms: Fever, headache, neck stiffness, and normal cerebral function.

Encephalitis: Inflammation of brain parenchyma, often viral in origin (e.g., herpes simplex virus).

Symptoms: Fever, altered mental status, seizures, and focal neurological deficits.

Chapter 25
Tetanus

Introduction

Tetanus is a life-threatening neurological disorder caused by the toxin produced by Clostridium tetani, an anaerobic bacterium found in soil and contaminated wounds. The disease is characterized by painful muscle spasms and rigidity, often progressing to severe autonomic dysfunction if untreated. The incubation period ranges from 2 to 38 days, with an average of 7–10 days. The severity of tetanus can be assessed using specific scoring systems, such as the Patel and Joag scoring system, which evaluates factors like patient age, duration of symptom onset, and the presence of autonomic hyperreactivity.

Severity Assessment Analysis

The Patel and Joag scoring system provides a structured approach to determine the prognosis of tetanus cases by assigning scores based on:

1. Age: Younger and older age groups tend to have worse outcomes.

2. Symptom Onset Duration: A shorter interval between injury and symptom onset indicates a higher severity due to more significant toxin dissemination.

3. Autonomic Dysfunction: Manifestations like fluctuating blood pressure, tachycardia, and arrhythmias reflect advanced disease stages and predict poor outcomes.

Patients with higher scores require aggressive management in intensive care settings, including mechanical ventilation and advanced hemodynamic support.

Therapy

Treatment involves immediate administration of tetanus immunoglobulin (TIG) to neutralize circulating toxins. The recommended doses are 500 units intravenously and 250 units intrathecally. Antibiotics are essential to control the bacterial load and include:

Crystalline penicillin: 20 million units intravenously every 4 hours for 10 days.

Metronidazole: 500 mg intravenously every 6 hours for 7 days as an alternative.

General Management

Airway Maintenance: Severe cases often necessitate intubation or tracheostomy to secure the airway and prevent aspiration.

Environmental Modifications: Patients are placed in quiet, low-stimulus environments to reduce spasm triggers.

Sedation and Spasm Control: Diazepam is commonly used in high doses, up to 500 mg/day, to control spasms and provide muscle relaxation.

Nutritional and Hydration Support: Essential for recovery, especially in prolonged cases.

Active Immunization

Because recovery from tetanus does not confer immunity, all patients must receive a series of three doses of tetanus toxoid. These doses should be spaced at least two weeks apart and administered at sites different from where TIG was given.

Tetanus Prophylaxis Protocol Analysis:
Proper prophylaxis is a cornerstone of tetanus prevention, especially in cases of injury. The protocol involves:

1. Clean or Minor Wounds: If the patient has received fewer than three prior doses of tetanus toxoid or if their vaccination history is uncertain, a single dose of tetanus toxoid should be administered.

2. Contaminated or Severe Wounds: In addition to tetanus toxoid, tetanus immunoglobulin (TIG) is recommended to neutralize any circulating toxin. For patients with incomplete vaccination histories, a full series of three doses of tetanus toxoid must be initiated.

3. Timing Considerations: Immunization and prophylaxis should be provided regardless of the time elapsed since the injury, as tetanus spores can remain dormant for extended periods.

This comprehensive approach ensures that patients are protected both in the immediate aftermath of injury and against future exposures, reducing the incidence of this preventable condition.

Conclusion

Timely assessment, management, and prevention of tetanus are critical to improving outcomes. By combining immediate therapy, appropriate use of immunoglobulins, and active immunization, healthcare providers can effectively mitigate the risks associated with this potentially fatal disease.

Chapter 26
Antibiotic Doses and Spectrum

Introduction

Accurate selection of antibiotics in the emergency department requires a thorough understanding of the causative pathogens and the antimicrobial spectrum of commonly used drugs. Empiric antibiotic therapy should be guided by the nature of the infection and the suspected microorganisms.

Antibiotic Doses and Their Spectrum

Crystalline penicillin is effective against a range of gram-positive organisms such as Streptococcus species and Listeria, as well as some gram-negative bacteria like Neisseria . It also covers anaerobes such as Clostridium.

Amoxicillin and ampicillin offer similar coverage but additionally treat Fusobacterium.

Cloxacillin is particularly effective against Staphylococcus aureus (methicillin-sensitive) and provides anaerobic coverage. Broader-spectrum agents like piperacillin–tazobactam and cefoperazone–sulbactam extend coverage to multidrug-resistant gram-negative pathogens such as Pseudomonas aeruginosa.

First-generation cephalosporins, like cefazolin and cephalexin, are effective against gram-positive organisms and a limited spectrum of gram-negative bacteria, including Escherichia coli and Klebsiella. Second-generation cephalosporins, such as cefuroxime, have a slightly expanded gram-negative spectrum, while third-generation cephalosporins like ceftriaxone and ceftazidime are more effective against resistant gram-negative pathogens.

Vancomycin and linezolid are potent agents for treating infections caused by methicillin-resistant Staphylococcus aureus (MRSA) and resistant enterococci. Linezolid also offers oral administration as an option for outpatient treatment.

Fluoroquinolones, such as ciprofloxacin and levofloxacin, provide extensive coverage of gram-negative pathogens, including Pseudomonas, and atypical bacteria like Legionella and Chlamydia.

Macrolides like azithromycin and tetracyclines like doxycycline are particularly useful for treating atypical infections and certain gram-negative organisms. Both classes are effective against intracellular pathogens such as Rickettsia and Mycoplasma pneumoniae.

Conclusion

Understanding the dosing and spectrum of antibiotics is fundamental for effective empiric therapy. Proper antibiotic selection ensures targeted treatment, minimizes resistance, and improves patient outcomes.

Section 5
Toxicology

Chapter 27
General Measures

Introduction

A comprehensive history is essential in managing toxic exposures, especially when patients, such as children, suicidal adults, or individuals with altered consciousness, cannot provide reliable information. Inputs from relatives, friends, or rescue personnel often play a pivotal role. However, even seemingly credible accounts may be misleading regarding the timing or quantity of ingestion. Observing the patient's environment, including partially used medications or signs of drug misuse, may offer critical insights. Pharmacy and medical records can also yield valuable information.

Decontamination is a critical emergency intervention designed to minimize systemic absorption of toxins. Key methods include gastrointestinal (GI), skin, and mucosal decontamination.

Gastric Lavage

Gastric lavage involves removing toxic gastric contents by alternately instilling and aspirating small volumes of fluid. Its effectiveness diminishes significantly if performed beyond the optimal window of 1–2 hours post-ingestion. Hence, it should only be undertaken when airway protection is assured to prevent aspiration.

Indications

1. Suspected life-threatening poisoning when patient history is unavailable.

2. Presentation within 1 hour of ingestion for life-threatening toxins.

3. Poisoning by anticholinergic drugs within 4 hours.

4. Sustained-release toxic drug ingestion.

5. Salicylate poisoning presented within 12 hours.

6. Ingestion of iron or lithium.

Contraindications

Avoid gastric lavage in drowsy or unconscious patients unless airway protection is ensured.

Technique

Insert a large nasogastric tube (16F) and confirm its position through air insufflation and auscultation over the epigastrium.

Position the patient in a left lateral decubitus position to reduce aspiration risk.

Instill 100–200 mL of warm tap water via the nasogastric tube.

Aspirate and collect the fluid in a dependent container.

Repeat the process until the aspirate becomes clear, typically requiring 500–3,000 mL of fluid.

Activated Charcoal

Activated charcoal is a highly adsorptive material derived from pyrolyzed organic substances, treated to maximize its surface area. It binds toxins in the GI lumen, thereby reducing absorption.

Indications

1. Drug ingestion with significant potential for toxicity and adsorbed by charcoal.

2. Presentation within 1–2 hours of ingestion.

3. Drugs with enterohepatic circulation or delayed gastric emptying.

4. Controlled-release preparations ingested within 12–18 hours.

Dosage

Mix 50 g of activated charcoal with 100 mL of water and administer orally or via a nasogastric tube.

Multidose Activated Charcoal:
Repeated doses may be beneficial for specific drugs, including carbamazepine, phenobarbital, and salicylates. The dosage typically involves 25–50 g mixed with water every 4 hours.

Contraindications

1. Depressed mental status without airway protection.

2. Late presentation.

3. Suspected GI perforation or obstruction.

Chapter 28
Drug Overdose

Introduction

Drug overdose often stems from intentional acts, but accidental cases, particularly among children, are not uncommon. Co-ingestion of multiple drugs or alcohol complicates the clinical picture, making the history unreliable. It is crucial to search for discarded medication packaging or other clues near the site of ingestion.

General Management of Drug Overdose

1. Stabilization: Assess airway, breathing, and circulation (ABC).

2. IV Access: Establish intravenous access and initiate fluid resuscitation.

3. Diagnostic Evaluation: Obtain relevant blood tests, including drug levels if available.

4. Decontamination: Perform gastric lavage or administer activated charcoal as per indication.

5. Supportive Care: Provide symptomatic and supportive measures.

6. Antidote Administration: Administer specific antidotes when available.

Specific Overdoses and Their Management

Acetaminophen Overdose

Toxic Dose: >150 mg/kg or >7.5–10 g in adults.

Symptoms

Nausea, vomiting, anorexia, and delayed hepatotoxicity (24–36 hours).

Management

Perform gastric lavage ± activated charcoal if presentation is within 1 hour.

Administer N-acetylcysteine (NAC)

150 mg/kg IV in 200 mL of 5% dextrose over 15 minutes.

Followed by 50 mg/kg over 4 hours and 100 mg/kg over 16 hours.

Use vitamin K1 (10 mg IV) if coagulopathy develops.

Tricyclic Antidepressant (TCA) Overdose

Symptoms

Anticholinergic effects (e.g., dry mouth, dilated pupils), seizures, cardiac conduction disturbances (e.g., QRS prolongation >100 ms).

Management

Sodium bicarbonate ($NaHCO_3$) bolus for cardiotoxicity.

Fluid resuscitation for hypotension; glucagon infusion or vasopressors as needed.

$MgSO_4$ (2 g IV over 20 minutes) for refractory ventricular arrhythmias.

Intubation for respiratory failure.

Other Overdoses

Benzodiazepines: Flumazenil is the antidote, dosed at 0.2–0.3 mg IV boluses until the patient is responsive.

Beta-blockers: Address bradycardia with atropine and administer high-dose insulin therapy for myocardial depression.

Calcium Channel Blockers: Administer calcium gluconate and high-dose insulin therapy.

The described interventions underscore the importance of timely assessment and targeted therapies in managing acute poisoning and drug overdoses effectively.

Chapter 29
Insecticide Poisoning

Organophosphorus Compounds

Organophosphorus (OP) compounds are widely used insecticides categorized by their toxicity levels and applications:

1. High Toxicity: Includes compounds like tetraethyl pyrophosphates and parathion, primarily used in agriculture.

2. Intermediate Toxicity: Examples include coumaphos, chlorpyrifos, and trichlorfon, used for treating livestock pests.

3. Low Toxicity: Compounds such as diazinon, malathion, and dichlorvos, often utilized in household pest control and field applications.

Clinical Features of OP Poisoning

Key features include

SLUDGE/BBB: Salivation, Lacrimation, Urination, Defecation, Gastric Emesis, Bronchorrhea, Bronchospasm, Bradycardia.

DUMBBELLS: Defecation, Urination, Miosis, Bronchorrhea, Bronchospasm, Bradycardia, Emesis, Lacrimation, Salivation.

Neurological Manifestations

1. Type I Paralysis: Acute in nature.

2. Type II Paralysis (Intermediate Syndrome): Occurs 24–96 hours after exposure, characterized by proximal limb and neck muscle weakness, often evidenced by the inability to lift the head from the pillow.

3. Type III Paralysis (Organophosphate-Induced Delayed Polyneuropathy, OPIDP): Manifests

2–4 weeks post-exposure with distal weakness, requiring weeks to months for recovery.

Cardiovascular Manifestations

Approximately two-thirds of affected individuals experience QTc prolongation, ST-T changes, and arrhythmias, potentially leading to severe hypotension or cardiac arrest.

Diagnosis

1. Plasma Pseudocholinesterase Levels: A rapid and accessible diagnostic marker, though not always reflective of clinical severity.

2. RBC Cholinesterase Levels: More specific but less commonly available.

3. Caution: Factors such as liver dysfunction, pregnancy, or certain medications (e.g., succinylcholine) can lead to false low results.

Management of OP Poisoning

Treatment should begin based on clinical suspicion without waiting for laboratory confirmation.

1. Immediate Interventions:

Skin decontamination.

Airway protection as needed.

Gastric lavage if presented within 1 hour of ingestion.

2. Anticholinergic Therapy:

Atropine: IV bolus (2 mg) escalating every 5 minutes until atropinization is achieved (heart rate >80 bpm, absence of secretions, SBP >80 mmHg). CNS side effects may include psychosis.

Glycopyrrolate: Similar efficacy with fewer CNS side effects; administered in 100 μg boluses every 2–5 minutes.

Maintain atropine infusion once stabilization occurs.

3. Cholinesterase Reactivators (Oximes): Use remains controversial and is not universally recommended.

Organochlorine Compounds

These pesticides, such as DDT and related agents, are known for their neurotoxicity.

Clinical Presentation

CNS excitation leading to seizures, agitation, nausea, hyperesthesia, and tremors.

Management

Stabilize airway and manage seizures using benzodiazepines, phenytoin, or barbiturates.

Gastric lavage is effective if performed within 1–2 hours of ingestion.

Atropine is not indicated.

Carbamates

Carbamates, like organophosphates, inhibit cholinesterase but with shorter durations of action (typically less than 48 hours).

Clinical Presentation:

SLUDGE/BBB and DUMBBELLS symptoms are similar to OP poisoning.

Management

Atropine administration is effective but requires lower doses and shorter treatment durations.

Intermediate and delayed syndromes are rare in carbamate toxicity.

Pyrethroids

Derived synthetically from Chrysanthemum extracts, pyrethroids affect neuronal ion channels, leading to prolonged excitation.

Clinical Presentation

Type I Pyrethroids: Cause hyperexcitability and fine tremors.

Type II Pyrethroids: Associated with salivation, hyperexcitability, choreoathetosis, and seizures.

Management

Supportive care includes gastric lavage within 1–2 hours and seizure control with benzodiazepines.

Atropine is not indicated.

Paraquat Poisoning

Paraquat is a highly lethal herbicide known for its corrosive and tissue-penetrating properties.

Clinical Presentation

Early symptoms include painful oral ulcers, dysphagia, nausea, and abdominal discomfort.

Systemic toxicity leads to multi-organ dysfunction, especially pulmonary, cardiac, hepatic, and renal failure.

Management

There is no specific antidote. Supportive care focuses on addressing organ failure.

Gastric lavage is contraindicated due to the corrosive nature of paraquat.

Hemodialysis may help reduce plasma paraquat levels but offers limited mortality benefit.

By integrating timely interventions and supportive care strategies, the outcomes for insecticide poisoning can be optimized. However, early recognition and swift action remain pivotal in mitigating morbidity and mortality associated with these agents.

Chapter 30
Rodenticides

Introduction

Rodenticides are widely used across India, particularly in instances of deliberate self-poisoning. While anticoagulant rodenticides generally exhibit low toxicity in humans, phosphorus-based compounds are highly lethal.

Types of Rodenticides

1. Anticoagulants

First-generation agents: Warfarin, , and coumatetrally.

Second-generation agents (super-coumarins): Chlorophacinone, diphacinone, bromadiolone, difethialone, and brodifacoum.

2. Inorganic Rodenticides

Zinc phosphide, aluminum phosphide, yellow phosphorus, and thallium.

3. Other Rodenticides

Strychnine and cholecalciferol.

Anticoagulants (Warfarin, Coumarins, and Indandiones)

Anticoagulant rodenticides interfere with the hepatic synthesis of vitamin K-dependent clotting factors (II, VII, IX, and X), leading to mucosal or internal bleeding.

Clinical Considerations

Second-generation anticoagulants have prolonged half-lives, necessitating extended monitoring of prothrombin time (PT) and international normalized ratio (INR).

Certain compounds, such as brodifacoum, may delay PT and INR elevations for up to 48 hours post-ingestion.

Treatment

1. Prolonged INR without bleeding:

Administer vitamin K1 (10 mg IV once daily or 10–50 mg orally 2–4 times daily) until INR normalizes.

High doses (100–400 mg/day) and prolonged therapy may be required for second-generation agents.

2. Prolonged INR with significant bleeding:

Use vitamin K1 along with fresh frozen plasma. For additional details, refer to Chapter 70 on Anticoagulation.

Phosphorus-Based Compounds

Aluminum and Zinc Phosphides

Found in powder, pellet, or tablet form, these compounds release toxic phosphine gas upon ingestion or inhalation.

Phosphine inhibits cytochrome c oxidase, causing rapid-onset toxicity, often culminating in death due to cardiac arrhythmias or refractory shock within 24 hours.

Clinical Features

Cardiac: Impaired myocardial contractility, circulatory collapse, and shock.

Pulmonary: Pulmonary edema (cardiac or noncardiac in origin).

Hepatic: Hepatic necrosis and fulminant liver failure.

Hematologic: Disseminated intravascular coagulation (DIC).

Metabolic: Severe metabolic acidosis.

Management

Treatment is primarily supportive, but survival rates are low despite intensive care.

Correct electrolyte imbalances, particularly hypomagnesemia, to reduce mortality risk.

N-acetylcysteine (NAC) may provide benefit if administered within 12 hours of exposure:

Dose:

150 mg/kg in 200 mL of 5% dextrose over 15 minutes.

Followed by 50 mg/kg in 500 mL of 5% dextrose over 4 hours.

Conclude with 100 mg/kg in 1 L of 5% dextrose over 16 hours.

Yellow Phosphorus

Yellow phosphorus exists in two forms:

Red phosphorus: Used in matchsticks and minimally toxic.

Yellow phosphorus: A highly toxic compound found in rodenticides (e.g., RATOL), fertilizers, and fireworks.

Clinical Features

Toxicity progresses through three stages:

1. Initial Stage (First 24 hours): Local gastrointestinal irritation or asymptomatic presentation.

2. Latent Stage (24–72 hours): Asymptomatic phase.

3. Toxic Stage (>72 hours): Multisystem organ failure, including hepatic, cardiac, and renal involvement, leading to death.

Management

Supportive care is the mainstay, although outcomes are often poor.

N-acetylcysteine (NAC):

Same dosing regimen as for aluminum and zinc phosphides.

Vitamin K1: 10 mg IV administered immediately.

Liver transplantation: In severe cases, this may be the only definitive treatment option.

Chapter 31
Plant Poisons

Oleander (Nerium oleander) and Yellow Oleander (Thevetia)

Tamil Name: Arali
Toxic Components: The leaves, flowers, seeds, and fruits of Oleander contain cardiac glycosides such as oleandrin, , and thevetin.

Clinical Presentation:

Consumption of Oleander leads to poisoning with symptoms similar to digitalis toxicity. These include:

Gastrointestinal distress (nausea, vomiting, abdominal pain, diarrhea)

Restlessness and confusion

Hyperkalemia: This is the most dangerous complication, as it can lead to life-threatening cardiotoxicity.

Cardiac Symptoms: These include bradycardia, atrioventricular (AV) block, atrial tachycardia, ventricular tachycardia, or even ventricular fibrillation. Severe cases may progress to cardiogenic shock and myocardial depression.

Management:

1. Early Intervention (1–2 hours post-ingestion):

Perform gastric lavage, followed by the administration of activated charcoal to reduce absorption, and consider a cathartic to expedite elimination.

2. Cardiac Management:

Bradycardia/AV block: Administer atropine or initiate electrical pacing.

Ventricular arrhythmias: Treat with phenytoin (3.5–5.0 mg/kg IV, rate not exceeding 50 mg/min) or lignocaine (1 mg/kg slow IV bolus, followed by continuous infusion at 2–4 mg/min).

3. Hyperkalemia Treatment:

Correct hyperkalemia with insulin and dextrose and albuterol nebulizations. Avoid calcium gluconate, as it increases the risk of arrhythmias.

4. Hypokalemia Management:

Hypokalemia worsens the effects of cardiac glycosides, so KCl supplementation (oral or IV) should be given.

5. Antidote:

Digoxin-specific Fab antibody fragments have been used successfully in cases of Oleander poisoning, though they are expensive and not widely available, particularly in countries like India.

Oduvanthalai (Cleistanthus collinus)

Tamil Name: Oduvan
Toxic Components: Cleistanthin A and B are the primary toxic agents found in the leaves, which can be ingested fresh, as a paste, or in a boiled extract.

Clinical Presentation:

Poisoning with Oduvanthalai can cause a variety of symptoms, including:

Gastrointestinal Symptoms: Nausea, vomiting, and abdominal pain.

Cardiovascular Symptoms: Chest pain, dyspnea (shortness of breath), tachypnea (rapid breathing), bradypnea (slow breathing), tachycardia, and bradycardia.

Renal Failure: Acute renal failure with distal tubular necrosis is a serious complication.

Electrolyte Imbalance: Hypokalemia is a common and potentially fatal abnormality.

Management:

1. Early Intervention:

Perform gastric lavage and administer activated charcoal within 1–2 hours of ingestion.

2. Electrolyte Imbalance Correction:

Correct hypokalemia and other metabolic disturbances. Administer sodium bicarbonate to correct acidosis, and consider hemodialysis for severe metabolic acidosis.

3. Cardiac Monitoring:

Cardiac pacing may be required in patients with significant arrhythmias or prolonged QT intervals.

Datura (Datura stramonium)

Common Names: Thorn apples, jimsonweed, devil's trumpets
Toxic Components: Atropine, hyoscyamine, and scopolamine, which are anticholinergic agents that cause typical cholinergic symptoms.

Clinical Presentation:

Patients with Datura poisoning often exhibit the classic signs of anticholinergic toxicity, which include:

"Red as a beet": Cutaneous vasodilation.

"Dry as a bone": Lack of sweat (anhidrosis).

"Hot as a hare": Hyperthermia.

"Blind as a bat": Dilated pupils (mydriasis).

"Mad as a hatter": Confusion, delirium, hallucinations.

"Full as a flask": Urinary retention.

Management:

1. Supportive Care:

Most patients recover with supportive care alone. However, some may require antidotal therapy with physostigmine (0.5–2 mg slow IV push over 5 minutes), which can be repeated in smaller doses if necessary.

2. Monitoring for Cholinergic Crisis:

Physostigmine should be used cautiously, as it can precipitate a cholinergic crisis (e.g., seizures, respiratory depression, bradycardia). It is recommended only for:

Patients unresponsive to supportive care.

Those with tachydysrhythmias and hemodynamic instability.

Severe agitation, psychosis, or seizures not responding to benzodiazepines.

Strychnine (Strychnos nux-vomica)

Toxic Components: The plant's seeds contain strychnine and brucine, which are highly toxic alkaloids.

Clinical Presentation:

Strychnine poisoning typically manifests within 10–20 minutes of ingestion. Symptoms include:

Neurological Symptoms: Anxiety, mydriasis (pupil dilation), hyperreflexia, clonus, and muscle rigidity, particularly in the face and neck.

Seizures: The hallmark feature is the "awake seizure", where patients remain conscious during tonic-clonic seizures.

Severe Muscle Rigidity: This may lead to tachycardia, hyperthermia, rhabdomyolysis, and severe metabolic acidosis.

Respiratory Paralysis: The most common cause of death is respiratory paralysis due to the involvement of the diaphragm and thoracic muscles.

Management:

1. Muscle Relaxation:

Administer high-dose benzodiazepines (e.g., diazepam 5–10 mg IV or lorazepam 2–3 mg IV) to control muscle rigidity. This can be repeated every 15 minutes as needed. In severe cases, propofol may be used.

2. Airway Management:

Aggressive airway management is necessary to prevent respiratory failure. Intubation may be required in severe cases.

3. IV Fluids:

Administer IV fluids to maintain a urine output of at least 1 mL/kg/h to prevent rhabdomyolysis and acute renal failure.

4. No Role for Gastric Lavage:

Gastric lavage and activated charcoal are ineffective and unnecessary for strychnine poisoning.

Conclusion

Management of plant poisonings involves a systematic approach of early intervention, supportive care, and targeted treatment for specific toxic effects. Identifying the plant and its active principles allows clinicians to tailor therapy to the specific type of poisoning, enhancing outcomes for patients.

Chapter 32
Snake Bites

Introduction

India is home to approximately 60 species of venomous snakes. However, the majority of venomous bites are attributed to the "Big Four" snakes, for which polyvalent antisnake venom (ASV) is effective. These four snakes are the Indian Cobra, Indian Krait, Russell's Viper, and Saw-Scaled Viper.

Russell's viper is unique in India for being both hemotoxic and neurotoxic.

Cobra bites are typically associated with neurotoxicity; however, if there is significant local reaction at the bite site, it is more likely to be a Cobra bite.

Krait bites tend to be painless and commonly occur at night, particularly in people who sleep outdoors or on the ground. If a patient is found unconscious on the ground, particularly during the early morning hours, a Krait bite should be considered.

Other venomous snakes in India include the King Cobra, Malabar Pit Viper, sea snakes, and coral reef snakes.

First Aid

Immediate first aid is crucial following a snake bite. The following steps should be taken:

1. Tourniquet Application: Apply a broad tourniquet above the bite site, ideally above the joint, to occlude lymphatic flow. The pulse should still be palpable below the tourniquet, and you should be able to insert a finger under it.

2. Limb Immobilization: Splint the affected limb to prevent movement, especially if it involves the lower limb.

3. Avoid Cooling and Incision: Do not attempt to cool the bite site or make any incisions.

Examination and Investigations

The assessment of a snake bite victim involves identifying the fang marks and evaluating signs of envenomation. The presence of two fang marks generally suggests a venomous snake, while multiple fang marks may indicate a non-poisonous bite.

Neurotoxicity: Symptoms include neck muscle weakness (difficulty in lifting the neck), ptosis (drooping eyelids), and a reduced single breath count (normal is 20-30 breaths per minute). A decrease in the count is indicative of neurotoxicity.

Hemotoxicity: Look for signs of bleeding, including petechiae, hematuria (blood in urine), gum bleeding, melena (black, tarry stools), and hematemesis (vomiting blood).

Coagulation Status: Whole blood clotting time should be assessed by collecting 10 mL of blood in a glass tube and leaving it to clot by the bedside. If clotting takes more than 10 minutes, coagulopathy may be present.

Other Investigations: Conduct a complete blood count (CBC), assess electrolytes, creatinine, urea, and urinalysis. Coagulation tests such as prothrombin time (PT), activated partial thromboplastin time (aPTT), as well as creatine kinase (CK) levels and an ECG should also be performed.

Management

Management of a snake bite focuses on symptomatic treatment, monitoring, and the administration of appropriate medical interventions:

1. Pain Relief: Use analgesics for pain management, but avoid NSAIDs if hemotoxicity is suspected.

2. Antibiotics: Consider antibiotics to prevent infection, with a focus on anaerobic coverage. Amoxicillin-clavulanate is a good option.

3. Tetanus Prophylaxis: Administer tetanus toxoid or diphtheria-tetanus (dT) vaccine intramuscularly into the deltoid muscle.

Anti Snake Venom (ASV)

ASV is derived from hyperimmunized horses, whose blood is processed to produce refined and concentrated venom antibodies. ASV is most effective against the venom of the "Big Four" snakes.

Dry Bites: Most snake bites are "dry," meaning they do not involve venom injection. ASV should only be administered when envenomation signs are present.

Premedication: Premedication is not typically needed for most patients. However, for those with a history of allergic reactions to equine antiserum, premedicate with:

Injection of chlorpheniramine maleate (1 ampoule, slow IV) and

Adrenaline (0.25 mg IM) in cases of suspected anaphylaxis.

Dosage of ASV:

For hemotoxic bites, administer 8-10 vials of ASV diluted in 5% dextrose over 30 minutes. Reassess the patient's bleeding symptoms and clotting status 6 hours later. Additional doses may be required based on severity.

For neurotoxic bites, administer 8-10 vials of ASV in 5% dextrose over 30 minutes. Reassess after 2 hours, and if neurotoxicity persists, administer an additional 4-8 vials.

Management of Anaphylaxis

In the event of an early anaphylactic reaction during ASV administration, the following steps should be taken:

1. Stop the ASV Infusion immediately.

2. Administer Adrenaline (0.5 mg IM, 1:1,000 dilution) and Chlorpheniramine maleate (1 ampoule, slow IV or IM).

3. After 30-60 minutes, when the reaction has resolved, the ASV infusion can be restarted slowly.

Additional Management Considerations

Respiratory Failure: If respiratory failure occurs, mechanical ventilation may be required.

Bleeding Management: If bleeding persists despite ASV, send for fibrinogen levels and arrange for fresh frozen plasma or cryoprecipitate.

Shock: Shock resulting from myocardial depression should be treated with fluid resuscitation and inotropes.

Renal Failure: Renal failure secondary to rhabdomyolysis or shock may require hemodialysis.

Ptosis: Ptosis caused by neurotoxic venom can persist for 1–2 weeks, but if there are no other neurological symptoms, there is no need to continue ASV for ptosis alone.

Cost and Regional Variations

The cost of each vial of lyophilized ASV exceeds Rs. 650, so it is essential to use it judiciously. Most venom used in ASV production is sourced from the Irula Tribal Society in Tamil Nadu, who catch the "Big Four" snakes. Notably, the venom from Russell's Viper in North India differs from that in the South, which may affect the efficacy of ASV across regions. Although there is no conclusive evidence, smaller doses may be sufficient in Tamil Nadu.

Currently available polyvalent ASV does not offer protection against King Cobra envenomations, which are found in the Himalayan region, Eastern and Western Ghats. Monovalent antivenom for King Cobra bites is available in some areas.

Conclusion

Snake bites are a medical emergency that requires prompt assessment and intervention. Accurate identification of the snake and the appropriate treatment plan, including the judicious use of ASV, is essential for optimal patient outcomes.

Chapter 33
Insect Envenomation

Scorpion Stings

India is home to approximately 86 species of scorpions, with Mesobuthus tamulus and Palamnaeus being venomous. The venom from these species induces the prolonged release of acetylcholine and catecholamines, leading to initial cholinergic symptoms followed by adrenergic symptoms. Interestingly, species with milder venom tend to cause more localized reactions.

Clinical Features

Benign Stings: Most scorpion stings result in intense localized pain but show no further progression of symptoms.

Potentially Dangerous Stings:

0 hours: Mild pain, tingling, vomiting, and increased salivation.

4 hours: Autonomic disturbances (sweating, priapism, cool extremities, tachycardia, hypertension, myocardial dysfunction, arrhythmias, and pulmonary edema).

48 hours: Shock, which may lead to death if untreated.

Investigations: Blood tests (CBC, electrolytes, creatinine), and ECG should be performed.

Management

First Aid: Apply an ice pack to the sting site.

Benign Stings: Pain relief with intravenous (IV) or intramuscular (IM) opiates or a digital ring block with 2% xylocaine (without adrenaline).

Vaccination: Administer the diphtheria-tetanus (dT) toxoid IM if the patient is not adequately vaccinated.

Antibiotics: Use antibiotics like cloxacillin or augmentin if infection is suspected.

Potentially Dangerous Stings:

Prazosin: 0.25 mg for children and 0.5 mg for adults every 3 hours until extremities warm up. Typically, 2–6 doses are needed. Start prazosin even if blood pressure is low. Noradrenaline infusion may be required.

Seizures: Administer benzodiazepines or phenobarbital.

Shock and Cardiac Failure: Treat with fluids and inotropes.

Life-Threatening Arrhythmias: Treat promptly.

Centipede Bites

Centipede bites are usually associated with local reactions, including pain, anxiety, vomiting, headache, and palpitations, though symptoms are generally mild.

Management

Pain Relief: Provide analgesics such as NSAIDs or opiates.

Local Treatment: Apply ice to alleviate discomfort.

Vaccination: Administer tetanus prophylaxis if not vaccinated.

Infection Prevention: Use antibiotics like cloxacillin or augmentin for signs of infection.

Allergic Reactions: Antihistamines can be used to manage local itching.

Bee and Wasp Stings (Hymenoptera Species)
Species like bees, wasps, hornets, and fire ants can sting humans when disturbed. Although most stings cause only mild, local reactions (pain, redness, and swelling), 0.3–3% of individuals may experience anaphylaxis, which can be fatal. After a bee sting, the venom apparatus often detaches and kills the bee, while wasps can sting multiple times due to their unbarbed stinger.

Management

Local Reactions: Treat uncomplicated stings with cold compresses.

Large Local Reactions: Use cold compresses, antihistamines (e.g., levocetirizine 5 mg PO for 1–2 days), and NSAIDs. Persistent reactions may require oral prednisolone (40–60 mg daily for 1–2 days).

Wheezing: Administer albuterol nebulizations.

Anaphylaxis: Treat with adrenaline, antihistamines, H2 blockers, and fluid resuscitation (refer to Chapter 3).

Stinger Removal: For bee stings, remove the stinger immediately with a 23-G needle or scalpel to prevent further venom release. After 5–10 minutes, stinger removal is less urgent, as most venom will have been released.

Wound Care: Clean and disinfect the sting site with soap, water, and spirit. Apply ice to reduce venom spread. If the patient is stable, advise the use of calamine lotion for local relief.

Other Insect Bites

Beetles, Caterpillars, and Millipedes
Certain arthropods like beetles and millipedes can cause severe burning pain, numbness, erythema, nausea, and vomiting. The treatment involves washing the area with soap and water, removing any spines or hairs using adhesive

tape, applying ice, and providing analgesics for pain relief.

Spider Bites

Most spider bites are non-venomous, though bites from species such as Loxosceles and Poecilotheria are reported in India. These bites typically cause erythema, pruritus, and swelling, with some lesions progressing to necrosis and eschar formation within a week. Management includes applying ice, antihistamines, and analgesics. For severe local reactions, antibiotics like cloxacillin are required.

Chapter 34
Substance Abuse

Opioids

Opioids are commonly prescribed for pain relief, especially in palliative care. However, both misuse of prescribed opioids and abuse of illicit substances contribute significantly to overdose cases. Frequently abused opioids include morphine, heroin, tramadol, methadone, and oxycodone.

Signs and Symptoms of Overdose

The hallmark symptoms of opioid intoxication include central nervous system (CNS) depression, respiratory depression, and miosis (constricted pupils).

Additional symptoms may include nausea, vomiting, orthostatic hypotension, localized urticaria, and bronchospasm.

Diagnosis is typically clinical, characterized by the classic triad of respiratory depression, coma, and miosis.

Management

Securing the airway and ensuring adequate breathing are critical.

Antidote: Naloxone reverses CNS and respiratory depression by competitive inhibition at the opioid receptor (OP3 receptor). Naloxone can be administered intravenously (IV), intramuscularly (IM), subcutaneously (SC), or intratracheally.

Dosing Guidelines for Naloxone:

Adults: Administer an initial dose of 0.4–2 mg IV bolus. Repeat doses of 0.4–2 mg IV may be given every 2–3 minutes until full reversal is achieved. The maximum total dose is 10 mg.

Children:

Under 5 years or under 20 kg: 0.1 mg/kg.

Over 5 years or over 20 kg: 0.4–2 mg IV bolus.

Additional doses may be required every 30 minutes to 2 hours, depending on the severity of the overdose.

Cannabis (Marijuana)

Cannabis contains over 60 cannabinoids, including delta-9-tetrahydrocannabinol (THC), the most psychoactive compound, as well as cannabidiol and cannabinol. Marijuana is often used recreationally by smoking dried flowers (joints or bongs).

Signs of Intoxication

Tachycardia, tachypnea, elevated blood pressure, conjunctival injection (red eyes), dry mouth, nystagmus, ataxia, and slurred speech.

Inhalation use may cause acute exacerbations of asthma, pneumomediastinum, pneumothorax, angina, or myocardial infarction.

Management of Acute Intoxication

Mild anxiety can be treated with benzodiazepines (e.g., lorazepam or midazolam).

Cannabis Hyperemesis Syndrome (abdominal pain, nausea, vomiting) is managed with IV fluids, antiemetics (e.g., ondansetron), and benzodiazepines.

Sudden onset chest pain should prompt consideration of acute coronary syndrome (ACS), pneumothorax, or asthma exacerbation.

Amphetamines

Amphetamines are commonly abused for their CNS stimulating effects, which can lead to complications such as vasospasm and intracranial hemorrhage, often due to hypertension.

Management of Acute Intoxication

Sedate agitated patients with benzodiazepines (e.g., diazepam 5–10 mg IV or lorazepam 1–2 mg IV/IM). Haloperidol (5–10 mg IM) can be used in psychotic patients.

Benzodiazepines should be used to control seizures.

If there are seizures or focal neurological deficits, a CT scan should be performed to rule out intracranial bleeding or subarachnoid hemorrhage.

For significant hypertension (diastolic BP >120 mm Hg), sedation may help. If not, treat it as a hypertensive emergency.

Cocaine

Cocaine is frequently abused and presents with symptoms such as seizures, hypertension, tachycardia, CNS depression, and cardiac arrhythmias. Chronic use can lead to paranoid delusions.

Complications

Cocaine use can cause angina, myocardial infarction (due to vasoconstriction of coronary arteries), cerebrovascular accidents (strokes), and psychotic reactions.

Management of Acute Intoxication

Sedate agitated patients with benzodiazepines to control seizures.

Manage hypertension as a hypertensive emergency and lower blood pressure rapidly with antihypertensive medications.

A CT scan should be performed to assess for intracranial bleeding if seizures or focal neurological deficits are present.

Sudden chest pain should be evaluated as a potential acute coronary syndrome.

Ecstasy (MDMA/3,4-Methylenedioxymethamphetamine)

Ecstasy, also known as molly, is a stimulant and hallucinogen that can cause life-threatening conditions such as cardiac dysrhythmias, acute liver failure, cerebral infarction, and hemorrhage. Severe hyperthermia (body temperature >40°C), metabolic acidosis, muscle rigidity, disseminated intravascular coagulation (DIC), and rhabdomyolysis are possible complications.

Management

Treatment is primarily supportive in a quiet environment, focusing on stabilizing airway, breathing, and circulation (ABC).

If the patient presents within 1 hour of ingestion, perform gastric lavage and administer activated charcoal.

Benzodiazepines can help manage agitation, seizures, or panic.

Initiate cooling measures for hyperthermia and monitor the ECG for potential arrhythmias.

Lysergic Acid Diethylamide (LSD)

LSD, commonly known as "acid," is a hallucinogenic drug that alters perception, thoughts, and awareness. Symptoms include pupil dilation, sweating, tachycardia, acute anxiety, depersonalization, and visual hallucinations. High doses can lead to seizures, focal neurological deficits (due to vasospasm), and coma.

Management

Treatment is largely supportive in a calm environment, ensuring stable ABC.

Benzodiazepines may be used to control agitation.

Gastric lavage and activated charcoal are not effective and should be avoided as LSD is rapidly absorbed through the gastrointestinal tract.

Summary

Substance abuse presents a significant clinical challenge, with each substance having its unique symptoms and treatment protocols. Early identification and prompt management, including the use of specific antidotes like naloxone for opioids and supportive care for other substances, are key to reducing morbidity and mortality associated with these substances. The management approach should be tailored to the substance involved, the severity of the intoxication, and the presence of complications.

Chapter 35
Miscellaneous Toxicological Emergencies

Corrosive Poisoning

A corrosive substance is one that causes damage to any surface it comes in contact with. The two main categories of corrosive agents are acids and alkalis, each causing different types of tissue damage:

Alkali ingestion results in liquefaction necrosis, where tissues break down into a liquid form.

Acid ingestion causes coagulation necrosis, leading to the formation of coagulated tissue.

Common Corrosives Include:

Acids: Sulfuric acid (car battery fluid), hydrochloric acid (toilet cleaners), nitric acid (metal cleaners), hydrogen fluoride (rust removers), acetic acid, phenol, and oxalic acid.

Alkalis: Bleach (hypochlorite), sodium hydroxide (lye, paint remover, drain cleaner).

Other Chemicals: Heavy metal salts (e.g., sublimate), formalin, iodine tincture.

Investigations:

Complete blood count (CBC), electrolytes, creatinine, liver function tests (LFT), ECG, rapid blood-borne virus screen (BBVS), chest X-ray, and soft tissue X-rays of the neck.

Management Guidelines:

1. If the patient presents within 24 hours of ingestion:

Do not administer gastric lavage due to the risk of aspiration and worsening of injury.

Establish intravenous (IV) access and initiate IV fluid resuscitation.

Remove contaminated clothing and irrigate ocular injuries continuously.

Administer pantoprazole (40 mg IV) and metoclopramide (10 mg IV) to manage gastric acid.

Provide adequate analgesia and refer to ENT for an assessment of the oropharynx and evaluation for upper gastrointestinal (UGI) endoscopy.

Endoscopy should be performed within 6–24 hours to assess injury severity and guide treatment.

If esophageal perforation is suspected, administer broad-spectrum antibiotics (e.g., clindamycin or ertapenem).

2. If the patient presents after 24 hours:

Endoscopic evaluation and intervention are less effective.

If no NG tube is placed, surgery may be required, including feeding gastrostomy or jejunostomy.

Follow-up and further endoscopy may be required based on injury severity.

Methanol Poisoning

Methanol toxicity typically arises from ingestion of illicit alcohol products. Methanol is metabolized into toxic metabolites, leading to metabolic acidosis and retinal toxicity.

Clinical Features:

Initial symptoms resemble alcohol intoxication (CNS depression, ataxia, nausea, and vomiting).

Severe toxicity includes CNS depression progressing to coma or seizures.

Symptoms of acidosis: Tachycardia, tachypnea, and hypotension, progressing to cardiogenic shock.

Visual disturbances such as blurred vision, photophobia, and potential permanent vision loss in about 25% of cases.

Management:

Supportive care: IV fluids to correct dehydration.

Correct acidosis: Administer bicarbonate.

Fomepizole: First-line treatment if available, to inhibit methanol metabolism.

Ethanol: An alternative treatment to inhibit the conversion of methanol to toxic metabolites.

Loading dose: Four standard drinks orally or 360–420 mL of 10% ethanol via IV.

Folic acid: To aid in formic acid metabolism.

Hemodialysis: Used to remove methanol and its metabolites in severe cases or renal failure, or if methanol levels exceed 50–100 mg/dL.

Kerosene Poisoning

Kerosene exposure can cause pulmonary toxicity due to aspiration, leading to chemical pneumonitis. Symptoms appear 1–8 hours post-ingestion, including breathlessness, nausea, vomiting, and abdominal pain. Radiographic findings may not become apparent until 72 hours later.

Management:

Do not induce vomiting or perform gastric lavage.

Provide supplemental oxygen if the patient shows signs of tachypnea or hypoxia.

In cases of acute lung injury, prophylactic antibiotics may be necessary.

Further management should be overseen by a medical specialist.

Inhalation Injuries (Carbon Monoxide Poisoning)

Carbon monoxide (CO) is a major cause of death in smoke inhalation. Inhalation injuries may also involve thermal damage, soot particle inhalation, and exposure to toxic combustion gases.

Clinical Features:

Symptoms of CO poisoning include confusion, altered sensorium, and physical signs like singed nasal hairs, hoarseness, and stridor.

Severe cases can present with seizures, syncope, arrhythmias, pulmonary edema, and acidosis.

Delayed neuropsychiatric syndrome can develop in up to 40% of severe cases, presenting with cognitive deficits, personality changes, and motor disorders.

Investigations:

Routine labs (CBC, electrolytes, creatinine, LFT), chest X-ray (CXR), ECG, arterial blood gas (ABG), and COHb levels.

COHb levels are not predictive of delayed neurological sequelae.

Management:

Remove from the source of CO exposure immediately.

High-flow oxygen via face mask or endotracheal tube.

Hyperbaric oxygen: This is a controversial treatment but may be considered in severe cases.

Airway management: Intubation may be necessary for severe respiratory distress or swelling.

IV fluid resuscitation: Based on burn severity.

Bronchodilators: Nebulized salbutamol if bronchospasm occurs.

Cyanide Poisoning

Cyanide inhibits cellular respiration by binding to cytochrome oxidase, leading to anaerobic metabolism and lactic acidosis. Cyanide is extremely toxic and can result in rapid death.

Sources of Cyanide:

Industrial exposure (plastics, metal polish, fumigation).

Plant and fruit sources (e.g., bitter almonds, peach pits).

Drugs (e.g., sodium nitroprusside).

Clinical Features:

Initial symptoms: Headache, confusion, tachycardia, and hypertension.

Severe toxicity: Bradycardia, hypotension, respiratory distress, metabolic acidosis, and possible organ failure.

Cyanide poisoning can present similarly to CO poisoning.

Management:

Immediate administration of antidotes:

Hydroxycobalamin: Binds cyanide more effectively than cytochrome oxidase.

Sodium nitrite and amyl nitrite: Induce methemoglobinemia, which binds cyanide.

Sodium thiosulfate: Facilitates cyanide detoxification.

Dosages:

Amyl nitrite: Inhaled for 30 seconds every minute for 3 minutes.

Sodium nitrite: 10 mg/kg IV.

Sodium thiosulfate: 50 mL of a 25% solution IV.

Hydroxocobalamin: 70 mg/kg IV bolus, repeat if needed.

Methemoglobinemia

Methemoglobinemia results from oxidation of hemoglobin, rendering it unable to bind oxygen, leading to hypoxia.

Congenital Methemoglobinemia: Caused by inherited enzyme deficiencies (e.g., cytochrome b5 reductase deficiency).

Acquired Methemoglobinemia: Typically due to exposure to drugs or chemicals.

Clinical Features:

Asymptomatic at levels <20%.

Early symptoms at levels >20% include cyanosis, lethargy, and tachypnea. At higher levels, respiratory failure and coma can occur.

Management:

Methylene blue is the treatment of choice for acquired methemoglobinemia. It reduces methemoglobin back to functional hemoglobin.

www.ingramcontent.com/pod-product-compliance
Lightning Source LLC
Chambersburg PA
CBHW071018240526
45469CB00006BD/1964